I0567305

Memory Improvement

How to Remember Anything &
Have Laser Sharp Focus to Impress
Anyone

*(Practical Strategies for Memory Improvement,
Brain Optimization and Accelerated Learning)*

Jason May

Published By **Elena Holly**

Jason May

Memory Improvement: How to Remember Anything & Have Laser Sharp Focus to Impress Anyone (Practical Strategies for Memory Improvement, Brain Optimization and Accelerated Learning)

ISBN   978-1-998901-98-2

No part of this guidebook shall be reproduced in any form without permission in writing from the publisher except in the case of brief quotations embodied in critical articles or reviews.

Legal & Disclaimer

The information contained in this book is not designed to replace or take the place of any form of medicine or professional medical advice. The information in this book has been provided for educational & entertainment purposes only.

The information contained in this book has been compiled from sources deemed reliable, and it is accurate to the best of the Author's knowledge; however, the Author cannot guarantee its accuracy and validity and cannot be held liable for any errors or omissions. Changes are periodically made to this book. You must consult your doctor or get professional medical advice before using any of the suggested remedies, techniques, or information in this book.

Table Of Contents

Chapter 1: The 'What' Of NLP

To positioned it truely, NLP is a systematic technique, related to the usage and optimization of three additives of the human machine, i.E. Neurology, linguistics and programming.

The NLP techniques were first done in 1970 with the beneficial aid of gents, going with the aid of the names of John Grinder and Richard Bandler. The number one interest of Neuro Linguistic Programming (henceforth known as NLP) is to tap into the hidden capability of the human thoughts, expanding its capacities beyond the traditional horizons.

It isn't any mystery that the human thoughts is able to storing and recording large portions of records, records and expertise, permitting the human kind to benefit goals effortlessly. However, this isn't pretty right, as set up by using the usage of innumerous humans excelling admirably particularly fields on the equal time as simultaneously failing in a single-of-a-type fields. For instance, it is quite a common phenomenon for a professional prodigy to have negative non-public individuals of the family, and a societal individual to lack the strength left to perform well professionally.

The sole reason of NLP is to channelize the energies latent inside the human mind toward a greater powerful motive, via deciphering the interplay a number of the idea approaches ongoing within the thoughts (neuro), the manner those notion strategies are expressed with the resource of approach humans (linguistics) and the reactions and conduct displayed in similar bobbing up situations (programming). By doing so, NLP enables making the final touch and fulfillment of dreams an easier venture.

We all understand, commonly our thoughts and moves range significantly. Our plans both are finished with bad execution, or we lack the punctuality to carry out them in time. Some steering is thereby required for you to synchronize our mind and actions with the aid of enhancing our behavior to match the conditions confronted. It strategizes our mind to live targeted on the venture at hand, in a worldwide wherein multitasking is speedy turning into the most huge fashion.

Chapter 2: About N-L-P

Before we can delve deeper into the packages, advantages and techniques of acting NLP strategies, we need to first have a test a few simple parameters and description a essential framework of the additives constituting this method making it lots much less complicated to understand the approach.

Neurology:

Neurology refers back to the working of the human concerned device. Before we interest on that, we want to first have a have a look at the components of the worried tool, mainly the critical concerned device- managing the direct acts of questioning, storing and compartmentalizing records and making plans and implementing moves- and the peripheral apprehensive machine, that is liable for the reflexive actions taken in unexpected, sudden situations, which do not require pre-processed mind.

Let us have a glance now at how the CNS talents. The CNS is the basis of all of a human's mind, judgment and perception. When in a state of affairs, our crucial concerned device analyzes the situation it finds itself in, and primarily based on both of the following it executes certain movements, making our frame reply mainly techniques:

• Based on previous memories: Experiences that are stored in our mind may be referred to as upon, to manual the mind in taking selections in comparable seeming conditions.

• Based on surrounding environment: In times in which there may be no previous experience of an event, the human brain inspires an answer this is deeply rooted inside the bringing up which we've were given long long gone through, and the environment the character has been subjected to.

As is evident, the whole lot from critiques to surroundings receives saved inside the human mind, and affects our manner of wondering. Due to this, people going via comparable conditions may additionally furthermore find out themselves using completely particular strategies on the way to pass about dealing with said state of affairs. This variance arises in particular because of the difference in perception.

It for this reason turns into essential if you need to compartmentalize and retrieve this statistics in an green, powerful way. NLP lets in us in doing just that.

Language:

Linguistics is the second parameter in NLP. In primitive phrases, linguistics is the take a look at of language. Here, it refers back to the medium adopted to hold our thoughts into actions and to express our perspectives. Though it could sound over-hyped, language might be the most important a part of having an effective and sensible goal attaining.

One of the number one drawbacks people face these days is that of miscommunication. They aren't able to explicit their perspectives in reality, or maybe they try, they emerge as speakme earlier than wondering. This regularly results in a blended reaction from the recipient of the message, and therefore hinders the overall performance of the thoughts of the sender. While this relates to out of doors verbal exchange, the same significance need to simply accept to inner verbal exchange, as there may be a continuous and consistent monologue ongoing within the history of the human mind, be it at the same time as desire making, or whilst comprehending a scenario. For this cause, inner conversation wishes to be clean, comprehensive and particular.

Programming:

Once the thoughts and our linguistics have been optimized to gain complete effects, they need to be coordinated collectively, as a way to educate the thoughts to art work inside the best possible manner, that is completed via programming, and having manage command over our mind & language.

The first step is to arrange our mind, feelings and mind, that allows you to growth the overall performance of the mind. As the announcing goes "A cluttered thoughts is the devil's workshop"! A litter inside the storage room of the frame can bring about undesirable, undesirable emotional outburst at inconvenient instances, thereby obstructing the overall performance of a person, in both expert or private fields.

It is proper here in which programming enables thru keeping on pinnacle of factors the emotions, disallowing them to intrude in a specific situation wherein it isn't required. It so takes place from time to time, that due to an overload of information the human mind can also sometimes get pressured on a manner to offer the proper information required in a situation. In this kind of case, programming allows with the useful resource of compartmentalizing and categorizing stored information, surely so facts retrieval can be optimized.

The Three Levels of Mind:

Our thoughts consists of three factors: the conscious thoughts, the subconscious mind and the unconscious mind. The conscious mind is the present day country of focus, of the surroundings and the statistics regarding it. This facts is pretty actually accessible for use via manner of the mind. The subconscious mind shops statistics which may be reached and retrieved with a few level of trouble. The information getting stored in the unconscious gets interpreted constantly thru the mind, however the mind isn't actively aware of this.

This concept will be better described through an instance. When we find out ourselves in a acknowledged environment, we routinely attain out without paying specific interest the environment, and conduct ourselves in a familiar way. Similarly, even as we communicate in our community tongue, the phrases come robotically, with out us having to place a similarly effort to conjure those phrases.

Chapter 3: The 'Where' Of NLP

High Stress Jobs:

Some professions together with medical jail, protection and so forth. Require excessive excessive ranges of strength and effort. Anytime an emergency case pops up, humans must file the least bit unusual hours of the day and usually be on their feet. Hence, sooner or later of downtime, it's far vital the ones people going for walks in the ones sectors keep a cool peace of mind, as lack of reputation on the gadget ought to have drastic, disastrous consequences. It is easier to lose focus because the thoughts is always in a rustic of over-work and tension.

In such times, even while the individual is resting, the subconscious thoughts exists in a rustic of anticipation, and this subsequently results in a highbrow breakdown among people going for walks in such situations. NLP permits to keep away from such undesirable situations with the useful resource of letting humans take manage of their personal minds.

It lets in in handling their ordinary responsibilities in a much smoother way, for that reason permitting them to coordinate their personal and expert lives higher.

Planning Jobs:

Jobs together with commercial enterprise employer, advertising and engineering which require severa making plans, accumulate an entire lot of blessings via using NLP professional minds. Having a vision and operating towards it, with fortitude, is the prerequisite for NLP, for this reason it proves useful to the people walking in these fields, as it's also a interest requirement in such professions. Long term initiatives require accountable desire making, that is one of the awesome superior by way of NLP.

Creative Jobs:

The important foundation of NLP is to interrupt preconceived notions thereby making the thoughts greater bendy. This first-class is available in on hand even as the

11

character is employed in a topic requiring innovative facts, like that of a painter, author or actor. When NLP is practiced, the thoughts will become willing to take risks and is likewise decided to convert those dangers into rewards. New thoughts emerge robotically at the identical time as all 3 degrees of the thoughts have been accessed in reality. Additionally, the translation of those thoughts does not require plenty of attempt, as in the case of untrained minds.

Social Life:

As crucial as non-public and expert existence can be, a person's social lifestyles topics in addition in in recent times's international. New people provide possibilities for brand spanking new critiques and exploring uncharted territories additionally boosts up our conceitedness. Different humans skip in terrific social circles, some huge, some not as a first-rate deal. But truly having a massive social circle does recommend that someone is handling it well. It is vital an amazing way to govern one's social circle inside the most green, however amiable manner viable, in a way that it interferes neither with one's personal lifestyles nor with expert.

A chaotic social existence is a bane in cover of a boon. NLP improves our verbal exchange, as it's far vital to voice our evaluations, however no longer on the charge of belittling the voices of others. The key's to strike a balance among our self perception and humility. NLP trains our mind to understand and maintain this experience of balance. Also, stereotyping and generalizing are of the biggest boundaries needed to be overcome on the equal time as constructing a healthy social existence. NLP imparts the character of open mindedness which lets in ultimately on the equal time as developing a healthy society.

Relationships:

Nowadays, relationships have become harder to govern, because of the humdrum of commotion inside the human thoughts, in addition to impatience and the tendency to surrender displayed with the aid of using most humans. This consequences in disastrous times of estrangement, divorces, separation among families and so forth. Oftentimes, all communications inside a family turns into null, as it high-quality leads to in addition misunderstandings and divide. NLP offers the masses required difficulty had to avoid such conflicts, to our lives, through urging the unconscious thoughts to interfere and submerge the urge to react aggressively. This can be done with the assist of NLP because it increases the rate of functioning of the subconscious mind. It trains the thoughts to have a say in important topics, apprehend the conflict and teaches it to simply accept that struggle isn't anything to fuss over.

Chapter 4: The 'How' Of NLP

Let us apprehend how NLP works, in advance than we have a look at the techniques to place into impact it. "Modalities" is the idea on which NLP is primarily based definitely upon. Modalities are the handiest form of every enjoy that we've in our lives. Representation of numerous physical and emotional senses like, seen, auditory, olfactory and gustatory senses are what modalities embody.

Depending upon the enjoy, modalities are further divided into sub-modalities. For instance, the sub-modalities for seen modality is probably brightness, coloration, clarity and so on. These sub-modalities coming together make a completely unique enjoy relating a specific experience.

To advantage a desired revel in, NLP works with the useful resource of converting the knobs on each sub-modality. By adjusting the quantity of sub-modalities, an contemporary revel in, assumed as consistent in nature, may be altered and perceived otherwise thru the brain. The changing of the altered enjoy with the actual one in our subconscious thoughts brings about a alternate in our movements.

This has an analogy to the strolling of track equalizer in our track machine. When the knobs on each frequency degree are altered, a genuinely one in all a kind fashion of song is produced notwithstanding the fact that the tune is identical. With the changed degrees of sub-modalities, a gift incident won't appear that terrible, than it did inside the past. Now, let's have a look at the steps to incorporate the NLP device in our lives

• First, assessment of your conduct sample is important. Your moves must be recognized properly beforehand, as NLP works on improving our actions. Taking test of ways you behave and react in a particular scenario is critical. It's better to preserve a document with you and jot down your actions in it as taking intellectual notes may be onerous and complicated after a element.

Every motion must be be aware down in element, collectively with the instances that delivered about it. Eventually, you can locate the manner your mind has set itself, a sample in your actions. The sub-modalities have to additionally be phrase down so you can regulate their degrees later. This will make your mind extra vulnerable to changes, liberating it out of this rigid shape.

• Here, you need a evaluation tool with recognize to which you can adjust your actions. For this step, be conscious down the activities of various people within the same situations as yours and then examine the two units of human beings. One doing higher and one doing worse than you in the field of state of affairs will assist you in making a particular column for each the units. Thus, helping you in evaluating your sports activities activities and moreover to research them for your assessment desk.

• After your observation and evaluation, deduce the facts to place into effect it to your lifestyles. As NLP is a reason orientated software program, set your desires earlier than you hold with this step. If a concrete intention isn't set at the same time as imposing it, you may will be predisposed to get greater burdened and there can be no effects. There are also chances of backfire if there may be pointless records muddle in your thoughts. So, make sure you have got a reason and artwork for this reason within the route of it.

• Next up is formulating a plan it truly is fine suited in your goals. Formulate the plan with the useful resource of making use of the behavior sample you noted down. To obtain the equal motive humans might likely have one-of-a-kind plans as each person behaves in a awesome way. This individuality is a key aspect of NLP. Find out the great and bad dispositions for your conduct with the useful resource of comparing your moves to the reference undertaking's actions. Keeping track of the change you are looking for to make and the extent of fulfillment in it, adjust your behavior therefore. Notice the changes that have took place via comparing your present day diploma of sub-modalities collectively together with your unique tiers.

• Once NLP is launched, music your improvement regularly. While imposing this system, noting down every progress and failure is critical as this will assist you in rediscovering your susceptible point and strength. Don't be disheartened effortlessly, as it's difficult to gain success inside the first attempt itself. Carry yourself notion by way of manner of perfecting your imperfections and applauding your self for each a fulfillment step that you have taken.

Chapter 5: The 'Why' Of NLP

In a world wherein multitasking and spreading oneself thin over a plethora of sports activities have come to be all of the rage, a software program like NLP, scientifically devised and examined for max effects, takes a the the the front seat with regards to self-improvement and development of 1's non-public brain and its capacities. In this financial disaster, we are able to discover how the techniques concerned in the NLP application can be remarkable carried out and exploited that allows you to benefit most blessings out of it.

Like most ideologies carried out in life, NLP practitioners don't forget that it is not WHAT you do this brings you fulfillment, however HOW you do it. Irrespective of the character of the way being finished, if finished with 100% typical performance ensures most efficient effects. Structure takes precedence over content material, and heavy recognition is laid on getting the project accomplished with minimum attempt, most performance and maximum extremely good time.

NLP teaches us to forestall demanding approximately earning profits, and alternatively divert all the strength spent into that within the path of more fruitful sports which incorporates long term planning, studying how money may be efficaciously invested, spotting and commencing themselves to possibilities and honing the abilties needed to find out fantastic investments.

The common man will recognize coins as being the first-class trouble in his existence, and could thereby deal with himself as a sufferer to the trap of cash. However, with the assist of NLP, we are capable of re-version our thinking so that we're no longer the victim on this rat race, and alternate a sure view we would preserve in our mind about ourselves. When we remember ourselves to be helpless, we're efficiently making sure in producing a thoughts-set that allows you to in addition promote and domesticate deep rooted emotions of helplessness, in flip exciting the unconscious's prediction of turning into helpless. This is what's known as a "vicious cycle".

However, while we study the requirements of NLP and channelize our thoughts to assume in a specific route approximately us, we learn how to control our perception technique. We also are able to absolutely recognize and recognize apparent cash making schemes, giving us the courage had to take the danger and consequently gain out for possibilities which cash can also offer. As NLP has designed the mid to expose any digging place right right into a mine of opportunities, three states of the mind consequently interact in ensuring that any selection taken almost about cash is applied with the very high-quality diploma of accuracy and precision, finally ensuring excellent results.

Seasoned veterans in the exercising of using the strategies of NLP to cash making confide that every one this is required is a trade from the terrible mindset related to coins, to a greater tremendous one, where new mind are embraced and welcomed. Negative beliefs and thoughts about coins want to be avoided so as for the NLP to paintings. Apart from this, it isn't quite a good deal seeing yourself in a rich position. It moreover enables to discover how human beings in influential and higher positions cope with their cash, further to the thoughts-set they undertake at the same time as dealing with cash. Money want to be appeared because the natural counterpart of building commercial enterprise corporation relationships and offering offerings to rich humans.

Once the human thoughts has been knowledgeable to understand cash as a stepping stone for success, and now not as a willing link to failure, it may be conditioned to investigate the excellent techniques and measures which can be taken to increase the money which one has in a single's hands into massive, great quantities. NLP moreover consists of a experience of being better capable of cope with earned coins. As is regularly the case, regularly individuals who earn huge quantities blow all of it away, via the usage of not being creative and practicing sustained spending. This is a downward spiral, which sucks out all enthusiasm and try needed to preserve a streak of positivity with recognize to coins making. NLP situations the thoughts to place into impact smart, properly perception out expenditure plans, and sporting out financial savings plans also becomes a miles much less hard assignment on the same time as coupled with the norms laid down with the resource of the NLP software program application.

Chapter 6: The 'Don'ts' Of NLP

Since there aren't any dangerous consequences to the NLP, it is anticipated that a few facet outcomes will present themselves over the route of the method. However, this is not the case. But some precautionary measures need to be taken but even as dabbling with NLP, which prevent the plan from going awry resulting in disastrous give up outputs.

• As the foundation for this system rests on the idea of assessment, it's far crucial to no longer flow into overboard through over estimating extraordinary people or undermining one's very personal capacities, as this consequences in a entire derailment of the purpose of this system. Holding oneself on a excessive pedestal can also have derogative consequences, as self-complaint is an essential feedback examine degree for any self-development scheme.

• NLP especially specializes within the control of feelings, and emotions via controlling measures. NLP allows in carrying out recognition and corporation, through controlling feelings and actions. However, this must finished inner limits, as a whole lack of feelings will make someone cold and insensitive and destroy one's individuals of the family and connections with humans. Overusing them or showing them in beside the factor conditions hinders development, and for that reason wants to be prevented. Be the boss of your thoughts, don't permit it boss you.

• Focus is high to getting outcomes out of this machine, so it's far vital to have a smooth goal in mind earlier than starting. Goals may be altered, as referred to in advance than, but too many changes can cause a burdened and befuddled thoughts. Once a aim has been set, try to interest on reaching the goal in its particular shape, in location of enhancing it in step with your whims. NLP is a scientific software program, performing on assessment of records, and as such must be approached as one.

• Do NOT anticipate effects at the first actual day of this device. The NLP software works in line with one's capabilities and the time taken for results to be exhibited varies from character to character, as each human is careworn out in some other way. Hence, raising your expectancies may additionally motive disappointments and a diminishing enthusiasm, which can show disastrous for mind control. Shortcut strategies and distractions want to be prevented in any respect fees, as this may nice similarly prevent the improvement of this system

Chapter 7: How Do Memories Form?

Our recollections do not actually form by means of danger. As we enjoy diverse things and preserve them in our recollections, there are quite some techniques that bypass on in our mind earlier than we are able to sincerely call those subjects as "memories."

In our mind, there are the so-referred to as synapses, which might be the connections amongst our thoughts cells. These connections are those in-charged inside the formation of reminiscences in our thoughts. All of the thoughts cells paintings with the aid of taking information from our reports, which in turn receives processed inside the brain and receives categorized amongst similar information.

Essentially, there are 3 sorts of human memory, especially the sensory memory, the short-time period memory, and the lengthy-time period memory.

All statistics that we attain with the usage of our vital senses, finally the term sensory. Once our senses understand some trouble—permit's say our ears pay interest a lovely melody—that information will then be forwarded to and analyzed in our mind. Our mind in turn will identify whether or not or now not that facts is thrilling enough as a way to keep it for your reminiscence. That is why songs which you like get stuck in your mind extra than the songs that you don't find out thrilling in any respect.

Meanwhile, our short-time period reminiscence (additionally called running memory) is that which our thoughts recollects briefly. For instance, if you take a look at the numbers 6528764 again and again, it'll in all likelihood be caught in your quick-term memory, which makes you trust you studied which you have already memorized those numbers; nicely, technically you possibly did, but this data most effective receives saved in your short-time period memory, and that is why you will be inclined to overlook it later on. According to Psychology Today, "Our short-term memory permits for brief don't forget and therefore has a tendency to be forgotten sincerely without troubles."

Lastly, all of the exceptional records that lasts in our reminiscence for a notably long term is that this is saved in our lengthy-time period memory. For instance, you still recognize that water is composed of atoms of hydrogen and one atom of oxygen despite the truth that the last time you have cited chemistry modified into years in the past. That is, of direction, because of the fact this information has been retained into your prolonged-term memory, which makes it last on your mind for an extended time than the range said within the preceding paragraph. It gets stored for your prolonged-term memory because of the fact you have got performed a memorization technique to don't forget this facts. Perhaps you normally use the term H2O in vicinity of water, so the facts absolutely receives stuck to your head. The idea is that the greater we retrieve recollections every so often, the greater it receives stored in our thoughts, which makes it less complicated to be retained in our extended-time period memory.

Moreover, there are vital strategies as to how our memories get saved in our thoughts. As cited in the preceding paragraph, our mind is the only this is chargeable for studying the information that our senses understand and encoding them into our reminiscence.

Chapter 8: Why will we forget?

Sheldon Cooper (executed with the resource of Jim Parsons in the hit TV comedy series The Big Bang Theory) is a person who has the so-called eidetic reminiscence, which makes him without hassle don't forget subjects as a whole lot as their minimal information—consisting of his buddy Leonard's (performed with the aid of way of Johnny Galecki) particular meal which he had days inside the past. Sheldon even has the capability to recite all of the gambling cards that they've inside the card recreation they name Mystic Warlords of Ka'a.

But we aren't Sheldon, of path. Unlike him who can without troubles endure in mind matters, we—as normal human beings—normally find it difficult to recall even small data, together with the suitable area wherein we positioned our vehicle keys or perhaps eyeglasses. In fact, we normally even need to write down the matters that we want to do not forget (thank goodness for the sticky notepads) just so we can't be capable of neglect it later.

As normal, there may be generally the antagonist or the villain in every story. As lots as it's miles crucial that we hold in thoughts the crucial subjects that we have to preserve in thoughts, we really maintain on forgetting them ultimately. Forgetfulness commonly makes our lifestyles less easy.

Now, you might be asking your self why Sheldon can maintain in mind matters and why you can't. You might likely have this unique query to your mind right now: "Why do I preserve on forgetting things?"

Four Theories of Forgetfulness

Researcher Elizabeth Loftus has upward push up in her studies on reminiscence with 4 sizable theories as to why human beings broaden forgetfulness. These theories consist of retrieval failure, failure to keep, interference, similarly to advocated forgetting.

1. Retrieval failure. Sometimes we have a propensity to overlook about a few detail because of the fact we are having a tough time to retrieve that memory. This instance is what we call due to the truth the retrieval failure. According to the decay concept, there may be a reminiscence trace this is common as fast as new recollections are stored in our thoughts. This hint will in the end fade and disappear, and—if no longer rehearsed and retrieved well—will then be long beyond all the time.

Retrieval failure frequently times gets improper with the so-called encoding failure. However, they are now not the dame. Encoding failure happens while you are not capable of properly encode the facts to the mind, this means that there may be no new memory this is long-established. You have been not capable of allow the statistics to enter your mind. Retrieval failure, however, is while you're able to enter the statistics in your brain however you aren't capable of hold in thoughts what that data is. You usually experience like that reminiscence is already at the tip of your tongue, but you may't in fact pull that facts out.

2. Failure to hold. Now, that's what we seek advice from because of the truth the encoding failure in which—as said earlier—you're no longer capable of store the records into your mind, it simply is why you just generally have a propensity to neglect it. Usually, this takes place when you are not capable of pay hobby or if there can be some element incorrect together with your senses (e.G. You've got problem in taking note of so that you can't keep in mind what music you've got truly heard) so you are not capable of permit the statistics input your mind.

For example, you noticed a female sporting a black shirt with a announcement written on it. You are able to do not forget that the female changed into sporting a black shirt because of the truth you allow that records for your mind. However, you couldn't be able to keep in thoughts what exactly become written on her shirt because of the truth you possibly did not interest extra on that element. You did no longer permit that facts to sink in to you, so that you can't undergo in thoughts what exactly that assertion have emerge as.

3. Interference. This concept of forgetfulness suggests that we, as people, have a propensity to miss topics due to the fact new statistics enters our thoughts. As our thoughts device new facts, the preceding one has an inclination to compete in addition to intervene with the new information. You are most probably to overlook subjects while the brand new statistics is much like the preceding ones, and your mind reveals it difficult to categorize it really is which. As a result, the ones forms of facts intrude with every precise, and the extra modern day one is much more likely to win.

There are sorts of interference, in line with Loftus. The first one is the proactive interference, which occurs on the identical time as the antique information in our thoughts makes it hard for us to permit new data in. Essentially, that is in which you beyond reminiscences prevent your mind to keep new recollections. On the opposite hand, in retroactive interference, it's far the state-of-the-art reminiscences that inhibit the antique ones from being saved in our mind. As new facts enters, there can be a excessive opportunity that you can lose your previously positioned out reminiscences.

Chapter 9: Seven Memory Facts

In this chapter, we can take a better check the seven exciting things that you need to recognize approximately reminiscences.

1. The hippocampus—that is part of our mind this is commonplace as a horse-shoe—is crucial in delivering statistics from our brief-term reminiscence to the prolonged-term. Once this vicinity gets broken, our brain may be now not able to enlarge new memories, that's what we recognize as anterograde amnesia.

2. The common sort of gadgets that our quick-time period reminiscence can shop levels from 5 to 9 first-rate. Moreover, many modern memory professionals don't forget that the real capability of our quick-time period reminiscence in terms of storing facts is round 4. That is why when you memorize a list of 25 phrases, you best keep in mind round five of them, due to the fact they get

stored for your brief-time period reminiscence excellent.

3. Our prolonged-time period memory shuts down at the same time as we're asleep. This is why whenever we're dreaming, we normally dream approximately the topics that we really noticed or idea approximately. On the opportunity hand, as soon as we awaken, we commonly generally tend to immediately forget about about what we have in reality dreamed about because of the reality our dream receives stored in our short-term memory as opposed to in our extended-term reminiscence.

four. Sleep deprivation usually effects in impairment in the functioning of our memory. When we get a excellent night time time sleep, our cells shape connections with every distinct. Moreover, the REM or Rapid Eye Movement sleep is related to the formation of our memory. This approach while you do not get enough sleep, your thoughts may also have a hard time forming new memory.

five. Brain connections are related to the formation of latest recollections. Many researchers propose that modifications in our brain neurons are commonly related to the creation of reminiscences. The connections amongst our nerve cells, which may be called synapses, permit data to tour from one neuron to every different. Changes within the synaptic connection in some areas of the thoughts (e.G. Hippocampus) are the ones which may be liable for mastering similarly to retention of new statistics.

6. There is a excessive opportunity that reminiscence failure may be inevitable as a person a long term. As a person reaches the antique-age, she or he has the tendency to have a decline near memory and particular capabilities. While there are a few elderlies who control to keep precise recollections as they age, professionals acquire as right with that genetic additives in addition to manner of life selections play a big characteristic as regards to sharp reminiscence.

7. You can beautify your reminiscence with the useful resource of performing some practices. While a few human beings obviously have sharp reminiscence, thru nature, we have the functionality to discover ways to enhance our memory. We virtually ought to observe a few memorization techniques further to make use of various useful gear and era as a manner to sharpen our memory. We will have a look at everything approximately this on the following part of this ebook.

PART TWO: IMPROVING OUR MEMORY

"It is all approximately the method and know-how how memory works."

Chapter 10: Mnemonics

Before we go to our essential discussion on this monetary ruin, permit me first provide you with this quiz: Memorize the seven important taxonomic tiers in Biology: nation, phylum, class, order, circle of relatives, genus, and species. Take be aware about the time that it'll take you to memorize those phrases. Now, strive memorizing this assertion: Keep plates easy or own family gets sick (Do now not mind the grammatical guidelines, despite the fact that!). Take phrase of the time this time, too. Now, which of these took you longer to memorize? Which one did you find out plenty less complicated to recollect?

Let us say that you have not taken Biology but, or you have got have been given already forgotten the topics that you have studied in you Biology elegance—due to the fact you have were given pretty a horrible memory that is why you're reading this ebook—it likely took you longer to keep in mind the taxonomic ranges than the hold-plates-smooth statement. That is because of the truth it's miles easier for your mind to technique statistics that looks to be greater acquainted to you than the facts that isn't.

Most of the not unusual topics that we usually tend to keep in mind effects are sentences (inclusive of the best given above), visuals, acronyms, or rhymes. When it involves memorization, we lease these items as a way to be lots much less tough for our mind to retain facts. This manner is what we call as mnemonics.

Mnemonic is a memorization method in which you relate records to visuals, sentences, rhymes, or acronyms to make that facts greater capacity on your thoughts to store. The fundamental function of mnemonics is to help our mind keep records resultseasily with the useful useful resource of diverting a large chunk of facts into extra practicable bits, at the way to be less tough a terrific manner to do not forget that data.

When you do mnemonics, you do no longer usually alternate what you are memorizing; you virtually change the manner you memorize topics. Essentially, mnemonics purpose to show the information into every other shape that allows you to our mind can without hassle hold as compared to the particular shape. As a depend of fact, even at the same time as you are nonetheless in the tool of moving information into a few different form, that records is already making its way to our lengthy-term reminiscence.

One of the generally used styles of mnemonics is the acronym because of the truth it's so an lousy lot simpler. It is at the same time as you take the first letter of each word until you provide you with a unmarried set of letters which you mind can preserve higher. For instance, at the same time as we have been little, we needed to memorize all the colorings of the rainbow, this is with recognize to the association of these colors. Because memorizing seven considered one of a type colours have become quite tough for us as little youngsters, we had been truely taught to undergo in mind the imaginary name Roy G. Biv, in which each letter of that call stands for each coloration of the rainbow. Instead of memorizing every colour, we simply use the acronyms of those phrases, i.E. ROYGBIV. And to provide ROYGBIV greater revel in, we recollect it as a call—Roy as the first call, G because of the reality the middle preliminary, and Biv due to the fact the very last name. That is because of the truth our mind can hold in thoughts topics that make experience to us much less difficult than those which do now not make feel the least bit.

When you use acronyms, you can additionally provide you with a phrase from the letters which you have. For example, you are trying to memorize the taxonomic tiers with the usage of acronyms, so you come up with the letters KPCOFGS. If you could take a look at it, it does no longer make experience in any respect. But if you could transform it right into a phrase, it is going to be easier so that you can make enjoy out of it because of the fact it is able to be a lot much less complicated on your thoughts to store. You may also look at it as KaPaCOFaGaS. While it does now not make experience technically, you an with out troubles keep it due to the reality it is pretty smaller than its real form. So in desire to memorizing Kingdom, Phylum, Class, Order, Family, Genus, Species, you without a doubt recollect the phrase Kapacofagas, that you comprehend stands for those taxonomic levels.

Mnemonics additionally can be applied in auditory form. Have you ever wondered why it's so a good buy an awful lot less tough at the way to remember song lyrics than, allow's say, all of the elements in the periodic desk? That is because of the truth track lyrics encompass melodies, whilst periodic table elements do no longer. It is the melody that without trouble receives stuck in our mind, which makes it much less complicated for us to consider the accompanying lyrics. The identical issue also goes when we first memorized all of the letters within the English alphabet. Twenty-six letters, which do now not make enjoy as a whole, had been quite hard to memorize. That is why we've got got the ABC tune wherein a melody became placed to the letters (the letters served because the lyrics). The melody of the song receives resultseasily retained to our thoughts.

Moreover, mnemonics additionally come in the form of poetry. Poem mnemonics additionally can be outcomes remembered when you consider that every line ends with a rhyme. An example of quick poem mnemonics is "I earlier than E except C, or at the same time as sounding like A in neighbor and weigh." As you could see, A and weigh rhyme with every distinctive, so it's miles less tough in case you want to maintain in thoughts that.

Although mnemonics are normally powerful, the effectiveness consistent with se nevertheless varies amongst unique age groups. How you redesign statistics from its specific form to a much less difficult one takes time and important assets. When it consists of younger kids, it's far better to use the only but modern-day devices to better engage their hobby and interest. Of direction, if they are paying interest, memorization might be less difficult. Moreover, kids will maximum possibly lose their hobby if what they're reading appears to be stupid and tough to recognize. Simple however revolutionary mnemonics encompass the ABC tune, it actually is attractive to most youngsters.

Chapter 11: Doing Associations

Another memorization approach is memorizing thru association. Basically, this approach, which is outwardly called because the Association Technique, is wherein we be part of new records with the ones which might be greater familiar to us, making it much less complicated for our mind to consider that records.

Experts liken our mind with pc file folders, because it collects new statistics and hold it with the antique ones, as long as the documents although in form with each one in every of a type. So even as you do the Association Technique, you absolutely hyperlink the ultra-cutting-edge facts, which you want to get saved in your mind, with the data this is already stored in your reminiscence, which in turn improves the risk of that information being retained.

The first thing which you want to endure in thoughts in associating new records with the antique ones is that the connection does now not always ought to make lots feel, and it does not need to be rational. The idea is which you truely ought to provide you with a connecting element, so you allow you to relate the trendy records to the vintage one.

When you've got information which you want to bear in mind, allow's say the word temporary because of this short-lived. You can translate this word into some detail— which does no longer always have to be a unmarried word collectively with this one— that is extra memorable to you, some thing this is greater acquainted with you. So you can divide the word temporary into, say, 3 splendid terms which can be extra acquainted to you: teach see(s) ant (teach see ant will sound greater related to temporary, but teach sees ant is extra grammatically accurate). So at the same time as train sees the ant and runs over it, that ant will die, of path, which makes it quick-lived.

Of path Association Technique does not best have a look at to memorizing clean phrases which includes temporary. It can accomplish that an awful lot higher than that.

For instance, you want to don't forget every digit of the pi (allow us to nice remember three.1416), you might imagine about it as a date, it certainly is March (representing three, being that it's miles the 1/3 month of the year) 14 (representing 14), 2016 (representing sixteen). Now, 3.1416 may also seem bit everyday to you, however three/14/sixteen or March 14, 2016 isn't, so that you can partner the modern-day records (3.1416) with the antique one (four/14/16).

Or in case you need to don't forget which you have a flight at 2 p.M., you may consider the aircraft with wings (of course, planes have wings). Two wings=2 P.M. Now, you have got simply related the ultra-modern facts (2 p.M.) with the antique one (plane's wings).

Moreover, affiliation technique additionally can be applied in remembering names. For example, if you meet someone whose call is Luke, you can accomplice that call with a few difficulty that is greater familiar with you, allow's say Luke Skywalker. So every time you could see that man or woman, you can take into account Luke Skywalker, so that you can remind you of his name this is Luke. Or in case you meet someone whose call is Gil, you can don't forget a hill. You can also even bear in mind it as "Gil went on a hill." So the subsequent time you need to recall his call, you may virtually must consider a hill, and you'll be reminded that his name is Gil.

See? It does now not even need to be that difficult to be able to bear in thoughts topics. Basically, the idea of the association technique is which you absolutely want to partner new information or reminiscence with the matters which you already apprehend so one may be much less hard in an effort to keep in mind them.

Chapter 12: Foods for Better Memory

I apprehend we have all heard about the pronouncing "you're what you devour." This is so cliché that on occasion we already neglect about what this actually technique. However, this applies honestly nicely. You are truly what you consume.

Food, as every person apprehend, deliver us one-of-a-type fitness benefits—for the purpose that we take the proper weight loss plan, of route. We apprehend thoroughly that proper vitamins brings approximately nicely health to us. However, it nevertheless looks like we do no longer apprehend exactly which weight-reduction plan we want to have. We commonly take suitable vitamins as a proper.

More than right frame fitness, there are a few factors that truely enhance our reminiscence. These are the food that play an vital role now not just in our not unusual health, but our cognitive well-being as nicely.

Generally, meals have an effect on the well-being of our mind because of the reality they consist of crucial nutrients that our mind desires so that you can characteristic well. Well, our memory is a big part of our commonplace fitness fame.

Aside from taking care of our body, we moreover have to take care of our reminiscence. We can achieve this with the help of our favorite friend—meals! Do no longer be afraid to trade your diet regime, though, due to the reality a outstanding weight loss program to your memory does now not genuinely have to be that complicated. In this financial disaster, we will take a closer check out which meals we need to encompass in our weight loss plan in order for us to beautify the functioning of our reminiscence. Before you even understand it, you're already eating healthful now not simplest for your frame, however for your mind as well.

1. Berries

Berries aren't exquisite delicious; they may be also accurate in your thoughts. That is because of the fact berries are rich in fisetin, a flavonoid which protects our thoughts cells from getting broken. Fisetin is manifestly discovered on strawberries further to exclusive types of stop end result and vegetables.

"Among girls who fed on or more servings of strawberries and blueberries each week, we noticed a modest bargain in reminiscence decline. This impact seems to be viable with distinctly smooth nutritional modifications," said Elizabeth Devore, a researcher who led this have a observe published in the Annals of Neurology.

According to the stated research, eating berries can maintain once more memory decline among older humans via approximately and a half of years. As every body realise, as someone some time, the tendency of memory loss receives better as well. Therefore, in case you maintain on ingesting berries, you can most probable postpone memory loss as you age.

2. Nuts

Peanuts do not precisely make humans clever consistent with se (opposite to what maximum oldsters assume), however as an alternative it makes our memory sharper. Generally, nuts—including almonds, walnuts, hazelnuts, and others—are a brilliant tool in boosting the functioning of your reminiscence.

Peanuts assist decorate your memory due to the truth it is wealthy in niacin, this is type of nutrients B critical for reinforcing the capacity of thoughts to absorb statistics further to do not forget antique statistics. More so, there are various research which have shown how powerful peanuts can be for our thoughts. In truth, those studies declare that peanuts are in truth useful in decreasing the opportunity of developing intellectual illnesses, maximum especially among adults who are vulnerable to having Alzheimer's similarly to Parkinson's illnesses.

In addition to that, walnut additionally has a immoderate DHA content material, that is notion form of Omega-three fatty acids. Omega-3 fatty acid is a nutrient that is desired via the thoughts for it to feature better.

three. Coffee

When you are pulling off a few all-nighter due to the truth you want to test (even though this is typically discouraged because of the truth as we have have been given stated within the previous financial ruin, sleep deprivation has a awful effect in your reminiscence), you are most probable to drink coffee so you will stay wide awake. However, espresso does not usually serve you by using maintaining you up all night time time; it additionally enables you beautify your thoughts's capacity to hold greater facts and recollections.

Some researchers from the University of Arizona did a take a look at on the impact of caffeine to human beings's memory. This have a take a look at has set up that caffeine consumption boosts our highbrow typical overall performance in addition to stimulates certain factors of our mind associated with our memory. Caffeine additionally controls some of our feelings and behaviors together with wakefulness, arousal, temper, and attention. In this take a look at, it changed into determined that adults who have taken 1/2 of of a pint of coffee honestly in advance than they took the memory take a look at displayed a substantial improvement of their average performance in comparison to those who did no longer.

However, usually hold in mind that too much of a few detail is terrible. Excessive espresso intake has a few aspect outcomes, too, which encompass shakiness and anxiety. So keep your consumption moderate.

four. Fish

Although occasionally fish get left out, they virtually bring about many wonderful effects to our properly-being, particularly to the fitness of our brain.

Researchers from University of Alberta studied the effects of DHA-rich meals to the development of our memory. In their take a look at, they have got determined out that having DHA-wealthy diet can upload omega-3 fatty acids to our mind. As what we've got got got mentioned in advance, omega-three fatty acids are vital in maintaining our mind wholesome.

"Supplementing your eating regimen with DHA, collectively with increasing fish intake, need to save you declining DHA tiers inside the brain as we age," said Yves Suave of University of Alberta.

Fish is a extraordinary deliver of DHA. So each time you consume fish, you furthermore mght keep extra omega-3 fatty acids on your thoughts.

5. Avocado

Aside from being a totally scrumptious fruit, avocado is also useful in keeping our reminiscence sharp. As a depend of reality, avocados are taken into consideration as an "all-spherical" fruit because it brings us numerous health advantages, together with safety in the course of stroke, thoughts damage, in addition to reminiscence loss. Just like different ingredients and fruits, avocados are a extraordinary supply of Omega-3s. Because of this, avocados assist in enhancing the manufacturing of blood in a single's mind, which in flip improves the functioning of the mind.

Adding avocado for your weight loss program won't hurt. You ought to have it in any way you need it. Avocados may be eaten as it's miles, you just ought to take the flesh and devour it. You can also create an avocado shake, which you high-quality must add milk and wonderful flavors for it to taste higher.

6. Eggs

Eggs are usually associated with lousy grades due to the truth its shape is similar to the variety zero. However, eggs don't have anything to do with getting horrible grades. In truth, mind in fact aids you to get better rankings whilst you remember that it is also this type of factors that assist you decorate your memory.

Eggs are an outstanding supply of choline, that is a nutrient acknowledged to be the mind's "reminiscence architect" as it allows inside the manufacturing of acetylcholine. Acetylcholine, then again, is a neurotransmitter in our mind that is right away concerned in our reminiscence. Choline is present in the myelin sheath, which in flip protects the mind's nerve fibers to useful resource in rapid transmission of electrical impulses.

7. Dark, inexperienced leafy greens

The subsequent time you see veggies for your plate, specifically the darkish and green leafy ones, do now not set them apart. These veggies, in truth, assist in the improvement of your reminiscence abilities.

Vegetables together with spinach, kale, similarly to broccoli are regarded to be wealthy in food regimen E and folate, which might be each vital on the subject of boosting our memory in addition to shielding our thoughts in widespread. Folate, for example, decreases the levels of homocysteine in our blood. Homocysteine is an amino acid that— whilst there can be a immoderate level— typically causes the death of our nerve cells within the mind. Therefore, while hormocysteine degrees are reduced, the possibilities of our nerve cells to die are also decreased.

Chapter 13: Ten Memory-boosting Guidelines

We have already mentioned within the preceding chapters numerous memorization strategies that you can do a good way to sharpen your memory. But doing those topics is not sufficient. There are but some steps which you need to do and specific concerns that you need to undergo in mind so you could have a much sharper reminiscence. In this chapter, we're able to talk about ten pointers which you need to keep in thoughts to enhance your memory.

1. Pay interest.

Before you even begin doing mnemonics or institutions, you will no longer get any in addition if you did not popularity on what you'll memorize in the first region. As what we have referred to within the preceding monetary disaster, there is the so-called encoding failure, in which we are capable of't bear in thoughts a detail as it became now not registered in our mind.

Always recollect that it's miles not possible to undergo in thoughts some factor which you do now not recognize. It is like looking for a report that does not even exist. Therefore, so as so that it will permit tremendous records to enter your mind, you honestly have to pay interest and cognizance.

For example, in case you are a scholar, you want to pay interest carefully on your instructor truely so you'll be able to take in the information. Likewise, if you are an employee, you have to be privy to what your boss asked you to do, so that you will not be able to forget about approximately it ultimately. Just keep in mind that paying interest is the first actual step that you have to do a great way to take into account matters.

2. Apply as many senses as vital.

Experts advise that when you use multiple of your senses, you may most probably to don't forget the statistics better. The more senses you operate, the greater you visualize and enjoy what you are gaining knowledge of, finally making it tons less complicated in case you want to memorize.

While it is important to be aware of what your professor is announcing in elegance, it's going to moreover be useful if you try to take down notes every now and then. Note taking, but, does not mean which you need to write down down everything that your instructor says. You fine ought to phrase the most vital things which you need to do not forget. Doing so makes use of no longer handiest your auditory enjoy but additionally your seen, considering that you may see the phrases and that makes it tons less tough that allows you to bear in mind matters (especially if you have photographic memory).

Moreover, if you are trying to memorize a speech, in desire to virtually analyzing them on the aspect of your eyes, you could moreover read them aloud. This does now not most effective help you exercising how you need to supply your speech, however also facilitates you memorize it resultseasily considering the fact that you could pay hobby it. Psychologists call this due to the fact the producing impact, wherein your memory is beautify as you are saying the terms aloud or typically you pay attention the phrases you are trying to memorize.

3. Avoid cramming.

This is the most not unusual mistake that many university college students, or maybe specialists, do. Many people count on that reading and doing paintings the night time in advance than the deadline is better than doing so every week in the past. However, numerous studies have confirmed in any other case.

Experts endorse that studying little by little over a number of times is better than studying the whole thing the night time time

time in advance than. That is because of the reality your mind is extra centered on what you are doing when you have masses of time, no longer like even as you are cramming and your brain is greater centered on wondering "I definitely have to complete this" in place of "I ought to analyze this."

Moreover, if you do now not cram, you've got were given enough time to divide data into greater feasible chew. But if you simply take a look at the night time time time earlier than, your thoughts might be too exhausted soaking up massive quantity of facts. As a cease end result, you can most possibly not endure in mind something or as a minimum most of what you've got were given studied the day after (given that most of them have been best stored on your short-time period memory).

4. Get enough sleep.

We have said in Chapter three that lack of sleep consequences in a horrific reminiscence. When you are disadvantaged of sleep, you will most probable broaden impairment in your reminiscence. I will repeat this: when we get a excellent night time sleep, our cells shape connections with every distinctive. The REM or Rapid Eye Movement sleep is related to the formation of our memory.

So make certain which you get sufficient sleep due to the fact this in flip improves your mind's capability to keep reminiscences.

five. Relate the state-of-the-art facts to the things which you already realize.

As what we've got were given referred to in Chapter five, associating new reminiscences with the antique ones assist you maintain more information. That is because of the reality you create a pattern to your mind that entails subjects which you already recognize.

When you are memorizing new matters, take time to relate these items to the information that you already recognize. Once you've got had been given already set up a dating among the vintage and the fashionable facts, there is probably an boom within the danger of you recalling the new facts.

6. Learn the way to visualize.

Visualization moreover allows you increase the threat of remembering subjects, mainly in case you consider your self as a visible learner. Visual newcomers are folks who are capable of go through in thoughts what they see a great deal less tough than what they pay attention.

When you are using textbooks, you want to moreover be aware of the visuals protected, which includes pics, charts, graphs, and others. This does no longer fine come up with a wreck from reading huge chunks of texts, however moreover permits you recognize most thoughts better, especially the precis ones. If there aren't any visuals included, you could opt to create your non-public. In a chunk of paper, you can draw, allow's say, a Venn diagram to demonstrate a few thoughts, or a mind map, or some issue suits your wishes and hobbies.

7. Make the most out of your brain.

Making your thoughts artwork is a top notch help while you are memorizing things. Just like our our our our bodies that want workout to get in shape, our brain additionally desires exercise to get healthier and higher.

You can try and do topics which might be out of your each day ordinary. For instance, you could carry out a touch simple mind bodily games, which consist of using your left hand (if you are right passed; left if in any other case) while you do matters which incorporates dealing with utensils on the identical time as eating, or typing collectively together with your mobile smartphone's keyboards. The concept of that is that you allow your mind get busy doing subjects which you are not used to, for this reason you workout your mind in absorbing new information.

8. Understand what you are trying to memorize.

When you are memorizing things, it's far very important that you apprehend the records in the first region. Psychology Today shows that you summarize a fabric the usage of your non-public phrases after which write or kind out that precis. You have to reorganize your precis on this form of manner that it'll likely be much less hard with a view to don't forget. "By manipulating the records in this manner, you're forcing your self to consider it actively," says Psychology Today.

Chapter 14: Know your Brain: Nature's most Sophisticated Machine

Do the subsequent duties one immediately after the alternative:

1. Visualize yourself smack in the middle of an area you'd want to be, like a cherry blossoms garden in Japan. Maybe a few area greater acquainted like your dwelling room at the same time as watching your favorite TV display. Create a concrete picture of the place to your mind, and hold it for a minute.

2. Listen carefully to the sounds inside the room which you're in right now. Concentrate. What do you pay attention? Stifled laughter? Barely audible conversations? Phones and fax machines ringing and buzzing?

three. Tap your palms at the table, in succession, a finger at a time. Then do a double faucet constant with finger. Then repeat in opposite.

four. Starting at a hundred, depend backwards with the resource of eight's.

5. Recall a past occasion from your beyond. The first time you drove a car. Your Mom cooking your chosen meal. Your first date. Try to endure in mind the whole thing approximately it: Who rode with you? What turned into the occasion? How involved did you get?

6. Pinch your self. Choose a smooth region to your forearm and pinch the smooth pores and skin tough enough to feel some pain.

Doing all six duties has activated thousands and masses of nerve cells on your thoughts to behave in nice coordination and timing which will produce the signals to, say, command your arms to tap in a particular series.

The mind has in no way been extra studied in records than right now. There are fairly-specialised machines that allow specialists to take actual-time photos of the residing mind at paintings.

A PET scanner might show that the simple challenge of tapping your hands in a predetermined series turns on the frontal cortex that makes you conscious that there's a task to do; the pre-motor cortex which deciphers the instructions; the motor cortex, which sends instructions to the arm, hand, and finger muscle corporations at the velocity of hundred miles in step with hour; and the cerebellum, which supervises the whole manner and makes positive which you perform the challenge on the subject of the floor of the table. The whole assignment takes some seconds to finish. Unknown to you despite the fact that, your thoughts has simply exhausted heaps and thousands of thoughts cells for that easy task.

The visualization exercising inside the first challenge turns on the visible cortex placed on the occipital lobe which sits at the decrease decrease decrease back part of the mind. Distinguishing person sounds round you devices off the auditory cortex inside the temporal lobe. Counting backwards via 8's works the prefrontal cortex, it really is accountable for planning and personality improvement. It is determined at the the the the front of the frontal lobe in charge of emotional expression, hassle fixing, language, judgment, sexual behaviors, and memory.

Remembering a reminiscence from your past turns on the hippocampus, that part of the thoughts involved in reminiscence plus the proper thoughts region that corresponds to the type of memory invoked, much like the motor cortex at the same time as remembering the primary time you drove a automobile; or the olfactory middle, whilst recalling the scent of your Mom's cooking.

In the final challenge, even as you pinched your arm, ache receptors in the pores and pores and skin sent alert signs and symptoms which were obtained through the use of the use of the thalamus which it then despatched to the cerebral cortex which finally decided the deliver and the intensity of the ache. The thoughts then initiates counteractions (freeing the pinch or shifting the forearm away) to save you similarly pain. In excessive instances, the mind releases endorphins, natural painkillers, which engage with opiate receptors to lower ache and promote a extremely good feeling.

The mind controls every trouble of your lifestyles, gambling an crucial feature in each emotion and idea that we experience. It is such an crucial organ that as a minimum 30,000 genes are committed to forming the mind. It weighs best 3 kilos but it consumes 20% of all of the gasoline that your frame takes in. That's enough strength to energy a mild bulb.

Your Brain on Metaphors

Metaphors are an powerful manner to make us understand mind ideas that we're capable of't experience right now. So, we are able to attempt to speak about the summary elements of the mind in greater concrete phrases just so we may want to make experience of the intangible skills of this very essential frame organ.

The mind is usually spoken about as like a laptop. If there's hardware and software application, the thoughts is often called wetware, and for precise purpose. The brain, like a laptop, gets enter (random quantities of statistics), strategies them, and springs up with outputs (relevant and usable statistics), before saving them in a record folder placed in its number one reminiscence for destiny use (reminiscence and don't forget). The thoughts can also additionally moreover behave like how a PC, on the equal time as online, have to do reflexive, actual-time processing; or, if offline, greater careful and calculated thinking. Unlike conventional pc structures which do sequential processing, which means they device statistics one after the other, greater current computers should now mimic the mind's capability to do parallel processing. The distinction comes with a pc being deterministic (the identical input will continuously produce the same output). The thoughts, then again, physical games "unfastened will." It want to respond and execute various commands from absolutely equal inputs. This function is what encourages the mind to growth creativity, form prejudices, and generate alternatives.

Chapter 15: How the Brain Forms Memories

Learning and forming recollections are complex methods. There are 100 billion neurons to your thoughts which may be continuously at paintings talking with thousands of various neurons at any given time. Neurotransmitters that adventure thru the synaptic gaps bind to specific receptor molecules placed within the neighboring neuron. Eventually, routine reports (stimuli) create synaptic connections and form a neuronal circuit or connections (pathway) it simply is surely reminiscence formation. When the equal stimulus takes place again, you react almost instinctively from reminiscence don't forget. This is the purpose in the again of the 10,000-hour precept, which states that 10,000 hours of deliberate workout is wanted to expose an athlete into a worldwide-class champion.

The mind sports activities involved in memory are complex and can be simplified as follows:

- Creating a memory

Our mind sends signs in a selected sample relying at the event we are experiencing. Consequently, connections most of the neurons, called synapses, are created.

- Consolidating the reminiscence

Memories which may be deemed insignificant are inevitably discarded. Those that want to be committed to prolonged-time period memory are consolidated for clean retrieval whilst wanted in a while. This way of sorting out reminiscences takes region all through sleep, while the brain recreates the events of the day.

• Declarative recollections are stronger for the duration of sluggish-wave sleep. Declarative recollections encompass real facts, preceding studies, and thoughts which have been intentionally accrued for sorting and storage.

• Non-declarative recollections, as a substitute, are greater brilliant sooner or later of fast eye movement (REM) sleep. Non-declarative memories embody procedural recollections, which assist you perform high-quality duties without aware cognizance of these previous memories.

Recalling the reminiscence

Memory recall refers to the subsequent re-having access to of facts and events from past reports, formerly processed and saved inside the thoughts. Simply located, it is what's called remembering. During recall, a pattern of neural connection receives activated in reaction to a comparable occasion. The thoughts most effective echoes it's notion of the occasion as although it's far taking vicinity in real time.

These replays, even though, are not strictly identical to the proper. The actual experience will usually be certainly one of a type from the memory recalled due to the reality it's far already mixed with new facts and antique memories, due to this remembering can be idea of as handiest a innovative re-imagination of the routine event.

Memories are not organized in our brains like books in a library. It's more like jigsaw puzzle quantities saved in separate elements of the thoughts related together with the beneficial aid of neural networks or circuitries. Remembering therefore includes revisiting the pathways usual for the duration of the previous experience. The power of those pathways will determine how short memory retrieval will rise up. Recall reloads an extended-time period reminiscence from garage into brief-time period or working reminiscence, wherein it could be accessed and used. It then re-stores the brand new memory from the experience into prolonged-term reminiscence for re-consolidation and strengthening.

Chapter 16: Techniques to Improve Your Memory

Memory lapses can be because of distractions, preoccupation, lack of popularity and weakened reminiscence muscle. There are numerous strategies to beef up your mind muscle agencies:

Give your thoughts a workout.

By the time you are an man or woman, your mind has already lengthy-established masses and loads of neural pathways vital in processing and recalling statistics rapid, solving effortlessly recognizable issues, and executing commonplace duties nearly right now. But sticking to those timeworn pathways, you're denying your thoughts the stimulation it desires to hold developing and developing. Your thoughts desires a few shaking up once in a while!

The "use it or lose it" principle famous in constructing muscular strength furthermore applies to reminiscence enhancement. The greater you state of affairs your mind to intellectual sports, the higher you'll be at remembering information. The excellent thoughts wearing occasions take you out of your normal and mission you to shape new brain pathways.

Good thoughts-boosting sports activities activities have the following elements:

• It introduces you to some factor new. An interest may be considered intellectually demanding, but if it's miles a few issue that you've already mastered, then it doesn't qualify as a splendid thoughts exercising. The pastime wants to be some thing which you haven't however tried and is out of your consolation quarter. It's your publicity to gaining knowledge of new topics and developing new abilties that ultimately decorate your brain.

• It's difficult and difficult. The first-rate mind-boosting sports ought to be difficult enough to call on your full interest. But as speedy as you've mastered the hobby, it received't require as an lousy lot mental attempt anymore and obtained't undertaking you as an entire lot as if you have been added to it for the primary time. For instance, getting to know to play a tough new piece of song on the piano counts. Playing a tough piece you've already memorized does now not.

• It's a talent you could enhance on. Search out sports that let you start at an easy degree and bypass up as your records progresses and your abilties beautify. When a as soon as difficult diploma starts offevolved to experience comfortable, that means it's time to transport at once to the subsequent degree of issue.

• It's pleasing. A revel in of fulfillment encourages the brain's getting to know gadget. It continues you engaged and concerned. As a result, you're more likely to maintain doing it and the extra the rewards you'll collect. So select sports activities sports that, at the equal time as hard, are however amusing and first-class.

Think of an hobby you've constantly preferred to attempt—learning how to play a musical device, talking a overseas language, gambling chess, or making pottery. So prolonged as an challenge maintains you engaged, they're sure to help you decorate your reminiscence.

Engage in physical exercising.

Mental exercising is essential for mind health mainly while coupled with bodily workout. Physical sports help your brain live sharp with the useful resource of growing oxygen deliver on your brain and decreasing the risks for problems which have an impact on memory retention together with diabetes and cardiovascular ailments. Exercise also encourages secretion of useful hormones that located strain and melancholy in test. Perhaps the maximum crucial advantage workout has on the brain is in neuroplasticity, thru stimulating new neuronal pathways recognized to improve memory formation and recall.

Physical Exercises which might be Good for the Brain

• Aerobic Exercises

In maximum instances, cardio sporting occasions which may be proper for your coronary heart are accurate on your mind as properly. Here's how cardio bodily sports benefit your mind.

• Aerobic bodily games repair broken mind cells thereby enhancing thoughts function.

• Cardio sporting events encourage secretion of the satisfied hormone dopamine. This makes you experience comfortable and happier. Regular exercising in ultra-modern alleviates signs and symptoms and symptoms of depression in human beings.

• Aim for 100 twenty minutes of slight cardio workout each week. You may additionally dedicate an hour swimming in the morning and some special hour within the night for dancing.

• Stick in your workout plan. Make it a addiction and a part of your day by day normal recurring. It may additionally help if you do it with an exercising buddy, so you may also moreover need to inspire every special.

• Don't push yourself on your limits. An excessive workout wouldn't do greater first rate in lowering your tension levels than an workout completed fairly. If you're simply starting, 1/2-hour of slight exercise will already do you wonders.

• Yoga

Yoga, even as coupled with meditation, permits interest and calm your mind. Needless to say, it reduces stress and maintains the mind in tiptop shape.

• It's moreover acknowledged to growth your life with the resource of slowing down mobile developing older.

• People who often meditate regularly say that they experience extra amazing, and that a happy disposition lets in them to deal higher with every day existence challenges.

• Walking

While strolling is the best and likely the least pricey exercise you may do, it is regarded to noticeably improve brain widely wide-spread overall performance.

• Regular walks permit one in each of a kind factors of your brain to speak with each one-of-a-kind. It has a few detail to do with the neural pathways which might be bolstered within the course of everyday walks. This enhancement of the neural connections makes you better at making plans, strategizing, prioritizing, and multi-tasking.

• Also, almost each person can experience a remarkable stroll, regardless of their degree of fitness or age.

• Jogging or Running

If you are a person with plenty of energy that desires burning, strolling or walking are the terrific sorts of exercise you may do at the begin of the day.

• A 15-minute run will assist lessen that more electricity to a point you need to get via your work for the rest of the day with out getting distracted.

• A brief run may assist you bring forth a hurry of the temper-booster hormone serotonin.

• Group Classes

For motivation and concept, bear in mind turning into a member of organization lessons. You'd continuously look ahead to jogging out because exercising turns into play more than a boring interest. Plus there's nothing more worthwhile than making new buddies.

For group activities, you can consider Aqua Zumba, Latin Hip-hop, Family Yoga, Tai Chi, or Group Cycling.

Chew gum at the same time as gaining knowledge of new topics.

Studies correlate chewing gum with extended coronary heart charge ranges ensuing to stepped forward circulate of oxygen-bearing blood into the mind. This in flip will increase hobby in the hippocampus, that part of the mind particularly chargeable for forming recollections.

Move your eyes sideways.

Make this part of your every day morning exercising. Move your eyes back and forth for 30 seconds. Why? In research, it have become determined out that horizontal eye movements make more potent the corpus callosum, a bundle deal of neuronal fibers that hyperlink the thoughts hemispheres: the progressive right thoughts and the logical left mind.

Clench your fists.

There became a have a take a look at achieved to decide how frame factors can be associated with how the mind features. It confirmed that clenching the hands improves a person's potential to memorize topics. Making a fist with the right hand aided in reading some factor, and switching to creating a fist with the left helped in undergo in mind.

At first, it appears farfetched that someone's fingers have something to do with reminiscence. The rationalization given emerge as that the hand-clenching stimulates the thoughts in a bypass-burdened out manner. Making a fist together together with your right hand activates the left issue of your mind; and the alternative takes area with clenching the left hand.

Use uncommon fonts.

Funky fonts sell better consider. There definitely became a examine that backs up this commentary. So if you surprise how making some factor difficult to check makes it plenty much less complex to keep in mind, proper right here's the reason: Think of the time you've skimmed thru text, were given to the quit, after which found out which you didn't pretty understand what the document said. The study defined that unusual fonts act like tempo bumps. Changing the font to make it greater tough to have a look at will gradual you down so you'd take a look at greater carefully, therefore improving your consider. A greater complicated clarification has some thing to do with self perception. When you come upon a writing that's tough to decipher, you end up a good deal much less confident of your ability for comprehension. As you sense stressful about now not know-how the cloth, you listen greater hard and go through it more deeply.

Doodle.

There's not anything like a smooth sheet of paper to lure the thoughts to doodle. Research suggests that doodling allows you let out your creativeness. Moreover, growing illegible drawings and writing down random mind encourages the mind to improve innovative questioning, to stay targeted and to maintain statistics.

Laugh.

Laughter allows lower levels of cortisol, the hormone related to pressure. When secreted in excessive tiers, cortisol is known to have an impact at the hippocampus, the short-time period memory consolidator, consequently impairing getting to know and memory.

Humor have to be included to your overall fitness plan for awesome extraordinary of existence whole of memories.

Start with those basics if you are searching out techniques to supply greater laughter to your life:

• Take your self a good deal tons much less severely. Share your embarrassing moments and learn how to chuckle at your self.

• When you pay attention laughter, gravitate closer to it. You be aware that you are usually satisfied to percent a few element funny due to the reality sharing feeds off the humor and gives you the threat to chortle all yet again. So in case you listen laughter, you knew that you just want to are seeking out it out and be a part of in.

• Spend time with playful, fun people. There are folks that snigger heartily at themselves and on the absurdities of lifestyles. They are brief to discover the humor in normal situations. Their great aspect of view and satisfied disposition are genuinely contagious.

• Surround yourself with pics that lighten you up. Put up a funny poster on your place of job. Set a pc screensaver that during no manner fails to make you smile. Display pix of you and your circle of relatives having amusing.

• Learn from children. Pay hobby to youngsters and apprehend that they may be the specialists on gambling, giggling, and taking life gently.

Practice accurate posture.

Posture is often omitted as a conscious expression of one's self. You won't be doing it right, suited statistics is it's feasible to make enhancements on the way you maintain your self, how it can ideally form your existence and destiny accomplishments.

In a chain of experiments, it have end up decided that frame posture may also have an effect on the preserve in mind of each wonderful and horrific memories. When sitting in a slouch and searching downward, have a check people located it a whole lot less difficult to remember helpless and terrible reminiscences than empowering and first-rate ones. When sitting upright with chins up, it's commonly smooth for individuals to preserve in thoughts optimistic reminiscences.

A right away posture generally improves memory because of the truth sitting upright encourages stepped forward blood glide and oxygen to the thoughts thru as tons as forty percent.

Feast on Mediterranean weight loss program.

Researches show that a weight loss plan of end end result, veggies, nuts, and fish (a whole type of meals this is common in maximum Mediterranean fares) isn't always handiest correct for your coronary heart however on your mind as properly. Vegetables and nuts are probable to fend off memory loss mainly in overdue adulthood. Fruits and Omega-three in fish are anti-oxidants an excellent manner to shield you from cognitive decline.

Take caffeine-wealthy liquids to enhance your memory consolidation.

Whether it is a cup of tea, a can of soda, or a mug of freshly brewed espresso, consumption of caffeine is the chosen energy booster for folks who want to evoke or live up. Studies have determined some other use for this stimulant: reminiscence enhancer. Although most of those studies located that caffeine has little impact in developing new reminiscences, the substance has definitely advanced reminiscence recall. Research has diagnosed caffeine to be a prime player in reminiscence consolidation, a technique wherein memories created had been bolstered number one to deeper level of memory retention and that consequently the substance is better ingested after getting to know a venture.

Be careful, no matter the fact that, to test if caffeine appears to intervene together along with your sleep at night time. If it does, reduce consumption or reduce it off altogether.

Meditate to beautify your strolling reminiscence.

The strolling memory might be likened to a chalkboard, in which you quick "write" bits of statistics like the place details of a place you're travelling for the primary time or names and faces of human beings you meet in an occasion. You hang immediately to the ones chunks of records till you're ready to type them into those that you permit circulate sincerely (because of the truth you haven't any use for them anymore) or the ones that you decide to prolonged-term reminiscence (for later take into account and use).

Working memory is the identical vicinity in that you do quick intellectual computations and preserve random info even as engaged in communication.

How does meditation help improve the running reminiscence? Studies display that regular meditation complements your capability to interest. Meditation will allow you to have greater control over your alpha rhythm, at the same time as your mind studies small easy bursts of strength sending you right into a kingdom of whole relaxation. This now not awesome improves your creativity however it allows you to clear out all distractions making it easy that lets in you to save crucial subjects to reminiscence.

Have a remarkable night time time's sleep.

Sleep is an essential problem in memory storage. It is at some point of gradual-wave sleep that the hippocampus replays all the sports that took place inside the course of your waking moments. Working below compressed time, it sorts via your studies as it documents away those which can be applicable on the identical time as discarding individuals who obtained't be big in the destiny.

Cultivate a amazing dozing dependancy via doing the subsequent:

• Commit to a ordinary sleep schedule via going to mattress at the same time every night and getting up on the same time every morning. Don't spoil your routine, even on weekends and holidays.

• Avoid TVs, phones, computer systems, and pills an hour before bed. The blue light emitted via method of those devices triggers wakefulness thru suppressing secretion of melatonin that induces sleepiness.

If you think that caffeine keeps you up at bedtime, lessen your intake or reduce it out absolutely. There are those who are overly touchy to caffeine that even coffee taken within the morning interferes with sleep at night time time.

Pay hobby.

Do you keep in thoughts that time while you had been making plans to shop for a pink Chevrolet and you determined that what catches your interest inside the course of your every day move back and forth are all the crimson motors plying your path. Pieces of statistics are committed for your reminiscence because of the fact you're inquisitive about them. When you extend a fascination for topics spherical you, you mechanically look at critical statistics and get them laser-etched in your thoughts.

Make time for pals.

We are social animals not intended to stay on in isolation. Relationships stimulate our brains. As a depend of fact, connecting with others might also very well be the extremely good shape of mind exercising.

Research shows that preserving worthwhile friendships and a assist machine are important now not only to mental and emotional health, but to thoughts fitness as nicely. In a observe finished via manner of the Harvard School of Public Health, researchers positioned that humans with active social lives had the slowest fee of reminiscence decline.

There are methods you can take gain of the reminiscence-boosting blessings of socializing, collectively with volunteering, turning into a member of a club, or accomplishing out to a person over the cellphone.

Concentrate.

There aren't any rapid-charging shortcuts to growing your consciousness. Today's global is so complete of distractions; not to mention the large volume of facts that we need to device every day. We absolutely simply can't type through all the records we're bombarded with day in and time out. Then there's the mission of determining what facts to keep and the manner to take into account them rapid. The mystery proper proper right here is to cope with large troubles first so your mind obtained't be pre-inquisitive about subjects which can unnecessarily clutter available mind garage place.

Use Mnemonics.

Another powerful tool in memorization is known as mnemonics. A mnemonics is a device (a rhyme, an acronym, an image, or a phrase) that will help you consider records or huge quantities of records.

There are superb kinds of mnemonic gadgets, namely:

• Visual photo. The trick is to accomplice a word or a call with a seen photograph this is colourful, colourful, and three-dimensional. Example: To maintain in thoughts the call

Robert Goldman, who works as an inspirational speaker, you could conjure an picture that you may partner with him, like a golden robot (which seems like Robert) this is talking non-forestall (his artwork involves talking.)

• Acrostic. Create a sentence in which the primary letter of each word represents the preliminary of what it is you want to bear in thoughts. Example: "My Very Excited Mother Just Served Us Nine Pies" in which the first letter of every word is the primary letter of the planets in our Solar System in order (Mercury, Venus, Earth, Mars, Jupiter, Saturn, Uranus, Neptune, and Pluto); or if without Pluto: "My Very Educated Mother Just Served Us Noodles."

• Acronym. An acronym is a phrase fashioned to symbolize the number one letters of all the phrases that make up a collection of key phrases or thoughts. Example: The acronym "HOMES" will help you undergo in mind the names of the Great Lakes: Huron, Ontario, Michigan, Erie, and Superior.

• Rhymes. Rhymes are effective techniques to take into account more common statistics and figures. Example: To consider which months have 30 days and which ones have 31, the subsequent rhyme is useful: "30 days hath September, April, June, and November. 28 days makes February first-rate, however in a leap 365 days it has 29.

• Chunking. Chunking is breaking aside a sequence of characters or an extended listing of numbers into greater capacity, easy to don't forget portions. Example: Breaking a ten-digit wide variety (say 5558765903) into 3 gadgets of numbers (555-876-5903) makes memorizing it hundreds less complicated.

• Method of loci. Also called the reminiscence palace, reminiscence adventure, or thoughts palace technique, this mnemonic tool works by way of the usage of way of imagining placing items you need to hold in thoughts alongside a acquainted course or unique locations in a familiar constructing (or "palace") or room. Example: For a shopping for list, photograph a puddle of milk in the entryway to your home, eggs sitting at the sofa, slices of bread scattered up the stairs, and bananas on your bed. Sing.

Music isn't best an top notch mood enhancer however an fantastic reminiscence device as properly. Singing sports activities the right side of the brain. Consequently, it makes you perform better at trouble solving. Ever phrase how you could with out trouble rhyme terms when you are singing them than whilst you are speakme them? This is because of the reality the music's melody has activated the pattern recognition capability of the right facet of your thoughts.

Stay Curious.

Always have appropriate urge for food for analyzing new subjects and an unquenchable thirst for cutting-edge facts. This is one of the best quantities of advice you may get to keep your brain in tiptop shape. Learning a contemporary idea from time to time heightens your recognition. Consequently, heightened attention results in statistics. It goes with out saying that the whole lot you understood, you'd consequences consider. For instance, understanding that the value of pi is the ratio many of the circumference of a circle and its diameter, you're great that it's far a regular rate because of the fact no matter the size of the circle, it's far continuously the identical shape. Interestingly, the rate of pi is an irrational range that is occurring and on. But you can memorize the primary 7 digits of pi by means of the usage of remembering this sentence: "How I desire I ought to calculate pi." Count the considerable type of letters in every word. It will provide you with 3.141592.

Read.

We can also gauge the reminiscence electricity of a person with the resource of the size of his vocabulary. Effective speakers will will let you realize that they do it thru studying as a exceptional deal as they're able to eat. If you don't have the high-priced of time, you can build your vocabulary via using the usage of analyzing one phrase each day. To improve dedication to memory, use your phrase-of-the-day at each possibility by way of the usage of the usage of the use of it to your interactions. That is without trouble 365 words a 12 months, more than enough terms to make a great have an effect on sooner or later of conversations.

Chapter 17: How Does our Memory Work?

Before leaping off to studying approximately the realistic reminiscence techniques, it's nice that you first understand how our reminiscence works so that you will understand how you could enhance it.

I. The Human Memory

The aroma of your mother's Sunday meatloaf, your first kiss, the unforgettable feeling for your bridal ceremony day—all our reminiscences make up a big part of what we're. How do you believe you studied you could navigate your manner through your condominium despite the fact that the lighting are grew to end up off? How do which corner to show to on the manner to your administrative center? All of this is due to our potential to do not forget.

When we speak approximately reminiscence, maximum humans ought to expect that it's miles just like every other part of the frame much like the eyes, nostril, or lips. However,

I'd consisting of you to recognize that reminiscence refers to a complex approach of remembering topics, like the examples I cited above.

In the beyond scientists pictured reminiscence as a tiny record cabinet located in a unmarried location of our mind. While others stated the reminiscence as a supercomputer that features a gazillion bytes of storage to keep records and immense tempo to retrieve them. Today, with the development of natural and physiological research, professionals had been capable of grow to be privy to that memory is more complicated than a filing cabinet, or possibly extra than a splendid laptop. Scientists now believe that our reminiscence is a method wherein specific regions of the thoughts play an crucial function in encoding, storing, and retrieving facts. It can be more as it should be described as a complicated net of connection (referred to as synapses) that grows more potent as we broaden and enjoy new subjects. You need to go through in mind that the ones connections come from the one of a type regions of the mind that makes up a single, rounded reminiscence of an person.

To supply an explanation for it in addition allow's take my instance in advance, as you are making your way to the administrative center, the reminiscence of the manner you energy your car comes from one part of the mind, the memory of the way you get from your own home to the workplace comes from each other, and feeling of caution while you're nearing a pedestrian lane or whilst crossing an intersection comes from a few different area of the thoughts—those type of elements coming from the ideal regions of the mind form a reminiscence: the way you energy from you home to the workplace.

II.Memory Processes

Now, how does the reminiscence artwork? How can our mind create and retrieve records?

i.   Encoding

The first and the maximum crucial step of the memory manner are encoding. It is the method in which our brain converts an experience or statistics right into a form (electricity pulses and chemical substances) that the brain can use. Encoding is our thoughts's capacity to create new reminiscence with notion through our senses—sight, sound, scent, touch, and taste. These perceptions adventure to the part of the mind known as the hippocampus that binds a majority of those into one unmarried revel in. These perceptions also undergo the frontal cortex and the amygdala in advance than it is correctly encoded with the useful resource of using the mind.

Our hobby or risk to the enjoy lets in our brain stumble upon whether or not or now not it receives encoded in our reminiscence or now not. This explains why we can with out problems memorize the matters that we are interested by.

ii. Storage

Depending on how the information is encoded (that is suffering from how vital we understand the facts is) the thoughts then shops the ones new facts into one of the 3 one-of-a-type "cubicles"—sensory memory, short-time period memory, and prolonged-term memory.

The sensory reminiscence can maintain impressions (the sensation of a hint, the sound of a automobile honking, the whiff of cologne, and plenty of others.) for pleasant a fragment of a 2nd to four seconds, counting on which experience come to be used to encode the memory. While the quick-term reminiscence allows us to maintain a nugget of information at a quick term. Our brief-term memory permits us to memorize phone numbers written on a billboard ad in advance than you write it on paper and it makes you keep in mind the query asked to you earlier than you get the hazard to reply. The quick-term reminiscence may be taken into consideration as an important degree due to the fact that is in which the mind determines whether or not or no longer the information can be discarded or whether or not or now not it ought to be transferred to the prolonged-term memory. The extended-time period memory on the other hand, is the garage that maintains crucial information that allows us in making selections and fixing troubles at the same time as the reminiscence is retrieved.

Experts offer an explanation for that these ranges of memory help us clean out all the records we come across every day to avoid records overload. Some statistics, because they may be no longer that critical, are handiest saved within the sensory or short-time period reminiscence, even as important statistics goes to the prolonged-term reminiscence.

iii. Retrieval

This part of the reminiscence manner happens on the identical time as you want to don't forget the statistics and also you consciously retrieve it from your prolonged-time period memory. Retrieval is a way that makes you recollect what you organized for the night time earlier than your big examination. This additionally enables you keep in mind critical dates in conjunction with wedding ceremony anniversaries, birthdays, and so forth.

00002.Jpeg

III. The Importance of Having a Great Memory

As I've said earlier, our memories are an crucial part of our lives—it makes us who we are. Our functionality to encode, maintain, and retrieve data are essential in our ordinary lives and maximum mainly even as we want it for making essential alternatives. Remembering our past opinions courses and lets in us in our gift and future endeavors. Our reminiscence allows us to research and endure in mind beyond mistakes in order that we're in a function avoid them subsequent time.

For students, having terrific memory is essential specifically once they want to recall what they reviewed to ace their checks. Good memory could also help profession-driven humans to overcome highbrow boundaries that may keep away from them from their achievement. Even complete-time moms may use a very good memory for them at the way to fulfill their obligations at domestic; even as older adults need to moreover artwork on having brilliant memory to live sharp even in their twilight years.

In brief, proudly owning first-rate reminiscence is important for everyone, old and young. And the first-rate thing is even individuals who are already in their senior years might also want to but paintings on improving their reminiscences. Continue analyzing and you'll find out how!

Chapter 18: Why can we overlook?

You in reality might not be conscious it, but forgetting matters can simply have an effect for your existence. Forgetting in which you placed your keys should mean wasted time seeking out it, forgetting about birthday anniversaries must endorse harm to relationships, lacking out on vital meeting schedules may also additionally mean an give up of the road on your profession. Given those situations, it's so apparent why you want to make a skip to beautify your reminiscence. But earlier than giving out the strategies on the manner you do this, permit's first take a look on the idea motive of forgetfulness. In this bankruptcy, you could find out the different motives why everybody forget approximately, you could studies what regular forgetfulness is and what isn't always. Also, you can take a look at the unique fitness situations that could impair reminiscence and you'll also studies if reminiscence loss is definitely an inevitable part of developing antique.

I. Common Reasons Why We Forget

In chapter 1, you placed out about the memory way this is encoding, storing, and retrieving. Some folks which are forgetful often assume that they actually have a awful memory. Assuming that you don't have any situations that could impair reminiscence, it's sincerely wrong to suppose that your whole memory method is failing you and making you neglect approximately subjects. Oftentimes, it's far simply one part of the memory way that has introduced on or is causing your memory lapse. There are multiple reasons why our reminiscence fails to remember information:

i. You didn't pay near interest

Do you want to apprehend why you preserve on forgetting in which you positioned your keys? More frequently than now not, people forget about wherein they left their keys is due to the reality they didn't in fact pay close interest to in which they placed it within the first area. Because of this, the mind didn't really encode something which means that that there may be no memory to retrieve.

ii.   There's an interference among memories

Another common reason why we forget about about approximately is while memories interfere or disrupt with every unique. This based totally on an concept referred to as Interference Theory in which one has a bent to neglect new or antique statistics because of the reality every reminiscences are interfering with every one in every of a kind. This is the reason why you preserve on forgetting your property's new mobile phone wide variety due to the reality your reminiscence stays stuck along side your antique phone variety (that is called proactive interference—at the same time as you neglect the trendy due to the vintage data). Or at the same time as you overlook about your business enterprise's vintage coverage due to the truth you're used to the new (this example refers to retroactive interference—

or at the same time as you overlook the antique due to the brand new statistics).

iii. Your mind didn't completely maintain the records

Another motive why people forget about approximately approximately is once in a while advantageous statistics encoded within the mind just become in the brief-time period reminiscence and no longer inside the prolonged-term memory.

Let's do an exercising to prove this. I need you to memorize this 12-digit significant range in 15 seconds, activity?

2,6,1,4,7,3,8,2,nine,5,7,1

Time's up! Without looking I need you to write down those numbers in a chunk of paper. Did you get it right? Don't worry if you didn't. That's because of the fact our quick-time period reminiscence can great preserve in mind seven digit numbers truly sufficient to memorize maximum phone numbers. (Did you understand that you could improve your memory and memorize as lots as 12 numbers? But we'll get to that later.)

iv. You are influenced to miss a reminiscence

This is applicable in particular to humans who've had professional traumatic activities to repress or certainly overlook about about unwanted memories. This idea is primarily based completely mostly on the Motivated Forgetting concept it is seen as a coping mechanism to suppress thoughts or reminiscences that reasons tension.

v. Our brain fails to retrieve statistics

Another commonplace reason why humans have "tip of the tongue" moments is on the identical time as their brains fail to retrieve the information stored in their memory. One concept that can give an cause of this is the Decay Theory which shows that after of the forgetfulness is even as a reminiscence fades with time. Remember about the connections in our thoughts known as synapses? These connections make bigger robust every time we maintain in thoughts statistics or an experience. In contrary, the connections decay or weaken greater time at the identical time as we don't usually retrieve the information.

II.   Aging and Memory Loss

Most humans take delivery of as proper with that memory loss—forgetting what you've got been meant to shop for within the grocery, failing to remember all the names of your grandchildren, or misplacing subjects, is an inevitable part of ageing. Some studies have examined that even those who are in their 20s are already experiencing cognitive deterioration.

But of direction, this isn't always absolutely real. Cognitive deterioration can be avoided in case you continually teach your mind as you age. If you don't do that, then you definately definately'll absolutely enjoy memory lapses even as you're vintage.

00003.Jpeg

Take be aware that our memory works greater like a muscle—the extra you use it and workout it, the stronger and sharper it receives. However while you forget about to use it, it deteriorates beyond regular time. This is one of the reasons why older people enjoy memory lapses, because of the truth they fail to constantly train their thoughts to stay lively. Other than this there also are a few physiological elements that heighten the threat of memory loss for older people. As we age, the hippocampus—the part of the thoughts this is accountable in encoding and retrieving data deteriorates when we age. Another motive of age-related deterioration is whilst the nutrient (protein) and hormones that protects the mind cells additionally declines whilst you age. But yet again, despite the fact that obtaining old ought to make you more liable to memory loss, it doesn't suggest that could't do some thing effective about it.

Now, which you apprehend that forgetfulness is a part of growing older, how do you recognize in case your forgetfulness is regular or a sign of a greater excessive scenario like dementia?

People who experience age-related memory loss can experience lapses occasionally however can despite the fact that bypass about their ordinary life. They can although make sound judgments, might also have problem in remembering the right time period to apply, however have no troubles in creating a communique, they'll be able to with out trouble navigate in familiar locations, and may notwithstanding the truth that capable of recollect the incidences in their reminiscence lapses.

On the opportunity hand, people who are displaying symptoms and signs and symptoms and symptoms of a more extreme situation that impairs memory loss exhibits trouble in performing even clean and everyday duties. You may additionally phrase them taking a bath or brushing their enamel severa times a day due to the reality they might't consider that they've performed it already. People who show off symptoms of these problems may additionally repeat their recollections in a communique or garble phrases even as talking with specific people. They may enjoy tension and can become disoriented while they are in extraordinary locations. Lastly, they make horrible judgments and might have problem making alternatives.

III.   Health Conditions that May Affect Memory

Besides age-related deterioration, there are awesome fitness situations which could impair reminiscence; some of the ones are:

1.   Dementia- refers to quite a few symptoms due to severa troubles wherein an man or woman's ability to expect and to create reminiscences declines because of mind cell deterioration. An person who's having problem in his quick-time period memory (can't consider what simply lately took place but can but keep in mind his/her youth years) is an early sign of dementia. Another commonplace signal of this condition

is someone's disability to discover the proper phrases in a communique, surprising modifications in mood, confusion, and problem of doing everyday every day obligations. According to analyze, oldsters which are at sixty five years and above are more vulnerable to growing this situation; but it is however now not a normal a part of growing older.

2.   Alzheimer's Disease- moreover known as AD, Alzheimer's is the maximum commonplace form of dementia that is affecting hundreds and masses of people global. In truth, in the United States on my own, it turn out to be cited that five million Americans have AD. Since Alzheimer's is a shape of dementia, an person with this situation may also even display signs and symptoms and signs and symptoms of having trouble with wondering, speaking, and remembering topics. They can also display symptoms and signs of persona modifications or sudden temper swings which might be a part of the scenario. Since AD is a cutting-

edge sickness, the signs and symptoms and signs and symptoms and symptoms of Alzheimer's will get worse beyond normal time. A person in the past due degree of AD may additionally moreover have trouble performing even smooth responsibilities like taking a tub, brushing tooth, or even ingesting.

00004.Jpeg

three.   Korsakoff Syndrome- notwithstanding the reality that now not considered strictly as a shape of dementia, an character with this sickness indicates the same symptoms and symptoms as someone with any sort of dementia. According to experts Korsakoff Syndrome is because of the shortage of thiamine (which allows the thoughts cells to supply strength) because of lack of nutrients and the inflammation of the belly's lining. Researchers have recognized extended length alcohol abuse to purpose this neurological illness.

4.   Amnesia- this term is used to outline situation in which an individual's reminiscence is misplaced or disturbed at a high-quality extent. Amnesia is visible to be due to numerous factors like head injuries, neurological illnesses or substance abuse. Experts classify Amnesia into types— anterograde amnesia or the issue in growing new memories and retrograde amnesia or the lack of a person's modern memory.

five.   Parkinson's Disease- in line with data this neurological ailment is affecting over six million humans global; typically aged 60 and above. This ailment is because of the deterioration of neurons in the substantia nigra, or the area of the thoughts that is responsible for motor manage. Some of the early signs of this illness are out of manipulate tremor, impaired stability, and speech modifications. Although this sickness mainly affects someone's motor capabilities, round 30% of humans that have Parkinson's boom dementia.

00005.Jpeg

If you believe you studied you otherwise you realise someone who well-knownshows the symptoms and signs I noted in formerly then possibly they're a candidate for this sort of situations. But of direction, you don't want to jump into conclusions proper manner. If you enjoy like your forgetfulness is apart from everyday, then I recommend which you are seeking out session at the side of your scientific health practitioner immediately.

Chapter 19: Brain Activities to Prevent Memory Loss

As I've said earlier, some aspect age you're, you can still discover ways to sharpen your reminiscence. Older adults, or maybe to folks that are in their 40's can sluggish-down the outcomes of age-related reminiscence loss or maybe beautify their reminiscence.

In 2008, psychologist Chandramallika Basak published a paper in Psychology and Aging on how a PC-endeavor "Rise of Nations" has advanced the cognitive talents of the 40 (older man or woman) those who took a part of the research. The recreation's purpose is to construct a city, feed the residents, train the city's army and expand the metropolis's territory—which required the members to make plans, multi-project, cope with ambiguity, and use their memory to gather the game. Half of the individuals received 23.Five hours training for the sport whilst the opportunity half of of did now not. After the have a test, the researchers have determined that the participants who had preceding education have notably superior their functionality to alternate in among obligations, beautify their reasoning capability and in addition to their reminiscence. It have become even cited that the members of the research have advanced brief-term memory seen cues. The check concluded that with normal education, even older adults can enhance their mind's functions which encompass trouble solving and reminiscence.

00006.Jpeg

Now of path, you don't have to play a video game to decorate your reminiscence. The crucial factor right here is that with non-prevent education and thoughts workout. Besides physical exercise, weight loss plan, and dealing with strain (which I will all speak in addition later), there are wonderful thoughts schooling techniques you could do to battle or cast off age-related reminiscence loss.

1. Engage in Brain Games

Because of vintage age, some seniors limit themselves to a daily everyday of searching TV, studying the newspaper, prolonged afternoon naps or really taking a short walk out of doors. However, sticking with this ordinary might boom their chance of age-related memory loss. Experts take transport of as proper with that as a way to sluggish down memory loss, it's critical that adults interact in sports activities that stimulates the mind.

Chapter 20: Techniques to Improve Memory

Have you ever at a loss for words why there are a few those who can memorize a exceptional amount of records? How can champions of reminiscence be capable of recollect names of 30 one of a kind people? How can they recite an extended grocery list virtually with the resource of searching at it for a couple of minutes? You need to realize the answer? No, it's now not because they've better degree of IQ. And No, they don't have greater memory storage of their head. All they did changed into educate.

Remember those years in the school room wherein you aced plenty of exams in fact with the aid of memorizing by way of the use of repetition or rote memorization? Learning with the useful aid of "rote" can be excellent in a few conditions however some of human beings argue that it isn't always relevant in lots of sports and it doesn't always assist a person have a look at and understand necessities in a deeper and extra complicated diploma. Most people try this method because of the fact they may be no longer familiar with the opposite techniques that paintings for one-of-a-kind types of memorization responsibilities. In this bankruptcy, you can apprehend and research extra approximately reminiscence strategies which may be basically strategies to results memorize nearly something. Learning how to utilize the particular forms of reminiscence structures will let you pretty improve your memory.

Memory champions spent years in their lives perfecting the method on a manner to enhance their reminiscence in wonderful stages. The desirable data is that you may additionally beautify your memory even if you're already a complete grown grownup. Even in case you obtained't be supplied as a Master of Memory, you could however use your reminiscence to work for you with the techniques that I will talk beneath.

Memory Techniques

Did you recognize that your thoughts is basically a filing cupboard for storing facts? A lot of human beings enjoy problems with remembering information now not due to the reality they may be no longer saved in their thoughts however instead they have got problems with retrieving statistics from memory. For you if you need to effortlessly keep in mind records, you need to learn how to installation your memory similar to how a submitting cabinet is classified, prepared and primarily based.

i. Visualization and Association

You can rent memory systems thru reading the artwork of visualization and substituting terms. Probably one the handiest and useful reminiscence method in keeping with many is the Visualization and Association (V&A) technique. Different humans recall matters through certainly one of a kind strategies: seen, auditory, or in writing. However, consistent with research maximum human beings are capable of memorize higher thru images (seen); and this approach takes gain of that.

The V&A method may be implemented through the ones simple steps:

Step 1:   Break down complex concepts via using way of substituting phrases

Step 2:   Take advantage of your brilliant imagination and redecorate the standards that you are trying to investigate into outstanding intellectual pictures

Step 3:   Think about all of the highbrow photos that you have created and hyperlink or   companion them with every different

Experts say that the important thing to memorizing some thing is forming a highbrow connection or associating the brand new statistics with records that you already apprehend. V&A is useful for people because we will be predisposed to be higher at remembering pictures than written or verbal data. The great component approximately this technique is that you could be as innovative, funny or revolutionary as you could as extended as it allows you bear in mind statistics higher. The institutions do not even have to make revel in. In short, the greater intellectual connections which you make among the vintage and new facts, the better the risk for bear in mind.

ii.   Mnemonics

You may additionally have in all likelihood used mnemonics inside the route of your life however did no longer realise it. Mnemonics are basically the short-hand for recalling remarkable bits of records with plenty much less attempt.

00009.Jpeg

For example, the mnemonic ROY G. BIV is generally used for remembering the spectrum of seen mild. You also can consider that this mnemonics stands for R-ed, O-variety, Y-ellow, G-reen, B-lue, I-ndigo and V-iolet.

There are really pretty some different mnemonic hints to decorate your reminiscence, a number of those encompass: Rhymes

If you need paying attention to track or making a song songs within the shower, you could use rhymes and lyrics to don't forget great types of records. You also can even turn whatever you need to keep in mind into a tune. For instance, if you are trying to maintain in thoughts the gadgets on your grocery listing, you could set up them in an order that rhymes:

Wheat bread

Peanut butter spread

Cream Cheese

Frozen Peas

A dozen eggs

Chicken legs

Your list can cross on and on as long as you can rhyme them.

Acronyms

Acronyms artwork by way of the usage of removing the first letter of the things that you are trying to memorize and then making up a word from them. If for example, the number one letters of the words does now not make enjoy, you may although positioned them collectively and memorize the random letters which you have mixed. HOMES is one of the maximum commonplace acronyms used to recollect the Great Lakes within the U.S. They stand for Huron, Ontario, Michigan, Erie and Superior.

Cross Words

You can also use pass phrases or acrostics to don't forget things less complicated. Acrostics are quite similar with acronyms but they variety in terms of creating a key-phrase. In acrostics, you need to take out every letter then create a phrase that corresponds to it.

Then, you string the phrases together to make a sentence that is simple to remember.

For example, in memorizing the natural groupings in taxonomy, in location of in reality making an acronym primarily based totally on their initials like KPCOFGS, you can make a sentence out of it like "Kids Put Candy On Four Gold Stars" to stand for Kingdom, Phylum, Class, Order, Family, Genus, and Species.

iii. Journaling

What higher manner to maintain and cherish reminiscences than writing them down on a magazine? If you're struggling with remembering terrific moments or facts of sports then keeping a journal may honestly help you maintain the ones accurate memories. Regardless of the way pinnacle your reminiscence is or the manner you enhance your episodic reminiscence, the records of powerful sports might in the end fade thru time. Fortunately, the solution to this is simple; you absolutely want to jot down them down.

Journal writing is one of the most effective techniques of improving your memory due to the truth you're actually recording the topics which you need to keep in mind 5, 20, or maybe 50 years from now. When you start developing the addiction of magazine writing, you will be extra familiar collectively along with your thoughts, feelings or feelings towards positive people, locations or sports.

iv.   Memory Exercises

Another effective method to decorate your reminiscence is thru automatically placing it to art work. If you really want to decorate your memory, you need to growth the highbrow effort which you located into impact each day. You can do that with the useful resource of way of carrying out plenty of reminiscence improvement wearing events. Here are a few guidelines to help you get commenced:

Cross Word Puzzles

You can bypass for the conventional pen and newspaper kind or you could trying to find online for pass word puzzles via your smartphone or pc. For instance, you can attempt to complete a puzzle each day every time you drink your morning coffee.

Memorize a listing and recite them backwards

If memorizing a listing of random gadgets comes smooth to you, then you want to degree up by recalling them in contrary order. You can do that at the same time as en direction to paintings or each time that you are idle. For instance, if you have placed the list of U.S. Presidents to heart, beginning from George Washington to Barack Obama, strive reciting it in reverse.

Perform Mental Computations

Now that we've clean get admission to to calculators on our cellular phones, we seldom perform highbrow computations. You can exercise your reminiscence through manner of absolutely acting smooth mathematical computations even as you are grocery shopping for. For example, you can get the walking standard of the fee of the grocery objects which you installed your cart.

v.   Capture Mental Snapshots

In my opinion, now not anything in fact captures a scene higher than the human eye. By consciously taking highbrow snapshots, you can improve your reminiscence in particular with reference to recalling events. They key to having a shiny mental picture and remembering it without trouble is by using manner of the usage of giving your complete interest it. By carefully focused on a few aspect is taking place, you are much more likely to take into account it better.

If you actually need an improved reminiscence, you want to located loads of strive into it. As you may see, you may strive an entire lot of techniques that will help you enhance your reminiscence each day. You have to consist of the ones memory techniques into your each day routine and located them to coronary coronary heart in case you want to achieve and enjoy the blessings of having a sturdy thoughts and a higher memory.

Chapter 21: 7 Lifestyle Changes to Prevent Age-Related Memory Loss

The reminiscence techniques and physical activities we included inside the preceding bankruptcy might no longer be as a whole lot effective in case you don't streamline your way of residing toward preserving a wholesome thoughts. According to experts, ideal components to prevent cognitive decline is retaining the mind energetic thru memory wearing sports and following a healthful manner of life. Listed below are a few way of existence adjustments you have to make as a manner to prevent age-related memory loss.

1. Get off the Couch- exercising

As I've stated earlier, regular sporting activities decreases the hazard or delays the consequences of reminiscence loss. If you've spent most of your life being a sofa potato, it's approximately time that you create a daily exercising normal. Even for the aged, a 30-minute stroll ordinary can not exceptional beautify the mind's fitness but additionally decrease the risk of sedentary lifestyle related illnesses in conjunction with excessive ldl ldl cholesterol, immoderate blood pressure, and weight issues.

"Physical workout has the top notch proof for maintaining memory and highbrow feature with developing vintage." says Dr. R. Scott Turner of Georgetown University Medical Center.

2. Get Enough Zzz's

Most people in recent times deprive themselves from getting sufficient sleep because of their busy time desk, tension, and masses of certainly one of a kind reasons. However, having an excellent night time time's sleep (7-9 hours) is crucial for an super thoughts function. That's due to the fact whilst we sleep, our mind is inside the tool of storing reminiscences which we will retrieve after a while. Also, researches have validated the dearth of sleep have to imply the slow increase of neurons that could motive hassle focusing, choice making and growing or recalling reminiscences.

three.   Quit Smoking and Regulate Alcohol Drinking

Did you understand that smoking can't best purpose issues on your lungs however can also have an impact on your mind's abilities as nicely? A have a look at in Northumbria University has established that folks who smoke in fact lose approximately 1/three in their reminiscence each day. While folks who already cease smoking were determined to retrieve reminiscence because the equal levels to those oldsters that during no way smoked in any respect. Also, smoking is hooked up to increase the risk of getting stroke which can yet again impair someone's potential to maintain in thoughts.

Alcohol abuse as a substitute can impair someone's judgment and memory. Long period of consuming can also growth a neurological illness Korsakoff Syndrome which impacts a mother and father' potential to do not forget. So the following time you're out together with your friends, recollect to keep it to the endorsed every day alcohol allowance (one bottle of beer for the women, and bottles for the guys)

four. Eat the Right Kind of Foods

Just like exercise, food regimen performs an vital characteristic in preserving the thoughts healthful. Foods which is probably rich in antioxidants, vitamins, and nutrients are those you need to stay with. Continue studying to the subsequent monetary catastrophe to discover the ten types of food that is proper for your thoughts's health!

5. Take Brain Supplements

Supplementing your thoughts with the right shape of vitamins and vitamins will double your opportunities of getting a healthy memory even as you age. Some of the nutritional supplements that promote thoughts fitness are creatine, caffeine to stimulate your brain's cognitive ordinary universal performance, flavanols,Omega-3 fatty acids, and Gingko Biloba that could be a well-known supplement in Chinese tradition.

6. Be Sociable

Some older adults may want to possibly sense like they have got had sufficient socializing of their manner of existence in order that they prevent exerting attempt to satisfy with one-of-a-kind human beings. However, research have verified that those who avoid social talents have extra danger of growing cognitive troubles. Staying linked collectively together with your family and buddies allows your mind to remain energetic and will prevent depression and pressure.

7. Manage Stress

Speaking of pressure, a test published in 2010 has validated that chronic strain need to truly have an impact on spatial reminiscence making it hard so that you can remember short-time period reminiscences. That's because at the same time as we're careworn, our frame releases a cortisol (a stress hormone) that weakens the thoughts's synapses within the a part of the brain pre-frontal cortex responsible in storing short-time period memory.

Chronic strain alternatively should without a doubt reduce your mind's neurons that make it tough in your brain to function well.

Find the premise cause of your pressure, exercising remedy, and workout are only some strategies on how you could manage your stress.

00010.Jpeg

Chapter 22: Feeding the Brain: 10 Foods that Boosts Mental Health

By now you realize that there are lots of factors that make contributions to age-related reminiscence loss like medicinal drug, alcohol abuse, smoking, lack of sleep, strain and greater. Besides adapting your manner of life with the pointers I referred to above, some unique manner for you to help combat memory loss and promote your thoughts's fitness is a healthful weight loss plan. Listed below are 10 forms of food if you need to maintain your mind sharp.

1. Fish Rich in Omega-three

Ditch ingesting beef or red meat and start whipping up dishes made with salmon, mackerel, and trout. These kinds of dishes are wealthy within the real form of fats known as Omega-three fat (in particular EPA and DHA) that are discovered to be useful now not extremely good for the coronary coronary coronary heart but moreover promotes a healthy mind feature as nicely. Eating immoderate DHA ingredients are visible to decrease the hazard of developing dementia, especially Alzheimer's illness.

00011.Jpeg

2. Whole Grain Foods

The mind wishes to burn power for it to characteristic properly. One of the healthiest belongings for thoughts energy is whole grain meals alongside aspect complete grain bread, brown pasta, wheat bran, and so on. These varieties of food is probably transformed by using using the body into glucose to be utilized by the entire body as strength. Whole grain foods are even secure for diabetics because of the truth those foods fall have low glycemic index which means that ingesting it'll no longer have hundreds effect on one's blood sugar degree. Be careful despite the reality that, some may additionally moreover mistake multi-grain labels to whole grain meals; truly recall to stay with the latter.

3. Blueberries

Blueberries are considered to be one of the international's top superfoods for the severa fitness benefits it gives. Don't allow the dimensions blueberries idiot you. Even in the event that they're small, blueberries are full of antioxidants that assist in stopping oxidative harm that would cause cognitive deterioration or dementia. It additionally consists of a phytonutrient referred to as flavonoids that protects the connections in amongst neurons and promotes the improvement of the mind's cognitive function at the side of reminiscence and studying.

One have a examine has proven that after the individuals (older adults that had a median age of seventy six) ate up 2 cups of blueberry juice (3/4 pounds a cup) in 12 weeks, showed sizeable tiers of enhancements of their cognitive take a look at rankings. This satisfactory proves that ingesting blueberries, regardless of what age you are, can beautify your mind's health.

four. Broccoli

If you hated your mom for forcing you to devour broccoli while you had been extra younger, now could be the time to discover ways to love them. That's due to the reality broccoli is filled with nutrients and minerals consisting of calcium, beta-carotene, iron, fiber, nutrients C, B, and K which might be all critical to combat the damaging free radicals and sell correct blood flow. It furthermore includes choline a micronutrient that promotes mind improvement and is visible to beautify the mind's capability to retrieve reminiscence.

five. Nuts

Consuming nuts, especially almonds and walnuts are showed to be useful for the mind's health. These nuts consist of Omega three and six fatty acids similarly to a whole lot of vitamins that improves the thoughts's skills. A studies achieved in UCLA confirmed that those who ate at least a handful of walnuts a day have extra ranges of cognitive characteristic (irrespective of age) than people who did no longer.

6. Beans and Legumes

These forms of elements also are rich in Vitamin B and omega fatty acids which is probably essential to keeping the mind's function in top form. Other than this, beans and legumes are fiber-rich and are categorised complex carbohydrates, which advocate they may offer the brain a consistent supply of glucose for use as gas for electricity.

7. Tomatoes

Tomatoes are known as a great supply of lycopene which permits hold a healthy mind. As an antioxidant, lycopene prevents the damaging effects of unfastened radicals that might cause cognitive deterioration beyond everyday time.

8. Spinach

Another antioxidant that promotes thoughts health is lutein it honestly is observed in spinach. Therefore consuming spinach will assist flush away toxin gather-up from that thoughts than can reason age-associated cognitive decline. A test at the Tuff University located that eating spinach in reality helped enhance the pupil's overall performance of their instructors. The examine located out that the scholars who ate more spinach had better scores of their exams than people who consumed a lot much less.

9. Avocado

Also considered as one of the healthiest food within the global, is the nutrient-rich avocado fruit. Like maximum mind meals, avocado is wealthy in Vitamin K and Omega 3 fatty acids that sell higher thoughts feature. It moreover has excessive levels of Vitamin E this is examined to beautify reminiscence, cognizance, and unique cognitive capabilities; and is also believed to contrary the outcomes of dementia, specially the Alzheimer's ailment.

10. Dark Chocolate

Yes! You can indulge into your chocolate cravings (actually stay with the darkish range) and decorate your mind's fitness. That's due to the fact eating darkish chocolate (encouraged amount is one inch square an afternoon) is examined to sell highbrow alertness, decorate popularity and attention. It moreover consists of flavanols which might be decided to increase the blood go along with the glide that is crucial for a healthy brain.

Include those fitness and nutritious meals in your every day weight-reduction plan and your mind will thank you!

Chapter 23: Memory as a Partner for a Student

Memory has extensive significance for college students. It is right now associated with the way they carry out from primary to university degree. From getting to know the alphabet to interpreting and memorizing extended formulas and sketches of sophisticated automobile models and plane fashions, reminiscence remains with us and become the stairs we use to gain higher tiers of studies and expert careers.

A student with terrible memory suffers from primary to college degree. She finds it tough to hold up with the rest of the elegance that would land her in waters. Most parents and instructors don't suppose memory is a essential trouble. They would snub the child blaming her sluggishness to be the real reason behind her beneath par general typical overall performance.

This economic smash interests at explaining to you what memory is and why it's far critical. It also can explain the signs and symptoms of terrible reminiscence so you are capable to test the lifestyles of these signs in memory and find out a probable answer for the hassle your scholar is going via.

What Is Memory?

The human thoughts is extraordinary at the same time as we accept as true with what it can gain. I was constantly interested by the way it labored and what it is able to gain. Just recollect the marvel of our questioning electricity and the manner we're able to recall hundreds of facts about a numerous variety of subjects. It is a complicated device. Memory is a wonderful cognitive way which permits us increase in lifestyles and society. It allows us to encode sure quantities of records that we achieve during a lecture at a university or college. It allows us keep and undergo in mind the records at a later time, specially in the path of examinations.

Memory performs a important function in shaping our lives. It lets in us to expand on the lower returned of analyzing from past and gift reviews. It is often a subjective and active tool of reflected photo of what has handed earlier than. For example, what you pay attention to for the duration of a lecture in a chemistry class remains for your memory. It additionally offers as a top notch deal as the present records in your thoughts.

Memory and studying are so deeply interconnected that we often confuse them with every unique, however they may be now not the equal in the eyes of specialists. Learning is commonly described as a device on the way to go away a long lasting impact on our persona; it shapes our mind and vision. Memory is our ability to keep in mind our past reviews. Take Emma for example, a student of a university. Emma is reading Chinese. She is going to the elegance, takes the lecture and is derived domestic to have a look at alphabets from a guide on Chinese language that she presented from a bookstall near her college.

Emma studies the book and memorize training to shop them in her thoughts for the long term. After that, she joins a collection of her classmates at a park in which she makes use of her reminiscence to talk the terms and terms that she had discovered. Memory plays an important function even as we are gaining information of recent subjects. It allows us to save new information and lets in us to preserve that statistics to recollect it at the equal time as we need to. We can say that reminiscence is the document that is left at the back of after an exhaustive getting to know technique.

Memory is proper now related to gaining knowledge of. Actually, both are interdependent on each unique. When Emma takes a new lecture on Chinese language, she connects the fresh facts to the statistics this is already stored in her brain at the equal topic. This affiliation of sparkling data to the triumphing records makes the reading method easy and smooth. If a college student suffers from a prone memory, his or her studying machine will genuinely be affected. On the opposite, if a scholar has a effective reminiscence, he or she can find out it masses less hard to maintain glowing facts. So, reminiscence has a deep impact on our mastering technique.

Though reminiscence has a reference to learning, it must now not be compelled with learning. There are sure techniques which are frequently at paintings within the human reminiscence.

Encoding: The very first of them is encoding. When Emma take lectures, her reminiscence converts the facts into a specific coded form that may be with out troubles stored inside the memory.

Storage: After the gaining knowledge of technique ends, our reminiscence stores the information in a selected part of the mind.

Retrieving: The saved records may be re-accessed from our reminiscence wherein we had stored it.

So there are usually 3 steps that our memory undergoes while we study new subjects. All the ones steps are part of the usual operational method. Generally, the general performance of learning is predicated upon on how green our encoding gadget is. Encoding is an energetic and selective machine that is relying on a huge variety of things along with the subsequent:

1. The first actual issue is the person of the content material which we're reading. Generally, it is based upon on the quantity of records that a pupil is receiving at some point of a class. The extra the quantity of data, the hard it receives to encode the records. The content material component is also stimulated by the usage of the level of company of the reading cloth. For example, if a scholar is reading a completely unique or a brief tale, she may be capable of without difficulty do not forget most components of the content fabric while she concludes. On the opportunity hand, if she is studying an precis element which include financial

statistics, she can discover it hard to encode hundreds of facts in a unmarried consultation. Another element that influences is the extent of familiarity with the content a scholar is gaining knowledge of. If she isn't acquainted with the difficulty, it's miles going to be hard for her to encode the records she is receiving. This is the reason why novices discover it hard at universities within the first few weeks. Another detail that impacts encoding new facts is how the content cloth material is mounted. Usually, the paragraphs at the beginning, center or at the end of a content material are without trouble encoded.

2.   The second thing is attached to the situations which play a function in encoding. It is likewise referred to as the environmental component. It is usually now not as crucial because of the fact the content material trouble is, notwithstanding the reality that it impacts our studying procedure. The climate wherein a pupil is living, the temperature of the lecture room, the extent of noise in the test room, frequency of interruptions, degree

of humidity, and conduct of the teacher are some environmental elements which play their element in memorizing information.

3.   The 0.33 is subjective element. They encompass powerful factors which incorporates the volume of fatigue, relaxation, u . S . A . Of health, interest in the problem and contemporary disposition of the student.

When the information has handed through the way of coding, it actions into the second one device of storing statistics. Storing is also crucial to the studying manner. If we fail to keep sparkling facts, we're able to be not able to recall it in the future. We can do plenty of factors with the saved facts. We can use it to form a hyperlink among smooth records and antique records, which makes the gaining knowledge of technique plenty less hard and fun.

Why Do We Forget and What Makes Us Forget?

This is a fact that we overlook even smooth topics. I agree that this will be one of the maximum troubling matters for someone. Most human beings get exceedingly irritated after they can't recall what that they'd memorized simply some time inside the beyond. We overlook everything together with names of human beings, their faces, and how and in which we met them. Perhaps, the maximum not unusual thing we forget about is the birthdays of our buddies and own family people. Come on, there's nothing excessive in forgetting the birthday of the only that you love. You can compensate it with a huge birthday celebration and an expensive present. The hassle begins offevolved offevolved at the same time as we start forgetting critical organisation meetings, names of our clients, and the amount of employer we do with them.

Have you ever perplexed why can we forget about approximately in the first region? There are nearly a thousand million neurons in our mind that permit us to carry out a bit outstanding topics which incorporates studying a couple of language and assemble topics which incorporates electric powered powered vehicles, robots, and rockets that could tear the outer environment and take us to place. I imply, this is great. On the only hand, someone's reminiscence is so strong that she or he will be capable of construct a rocket and a robotic, whilst some other character has to keep a listing of groceries written in his or her pocket because they outcomes overlook subjects (Cherry, 2019).

It takes place regularly while we forget about a few factor but keep in mind everything related to some other issue. There are sure motives why we overlook topics. Let's test some of them.

Retrieval of Information

Did you ever have a feel that a bit of facts has virtually slipped from your mind, leaving you surprised? It additionally takes area with humans that someone may additionally recognize a tremendous piece of information approximately but can't keep in mind it, or to position it this manner, can't hint it in their thoughts. The feeling of the existence of the information persists of their brain. The failure to retrieve a memory is every other purpose of forgetfulness.

One feasible motive for failure to retrieve data is known as the decay concept. The advocates of this concept say that our reminiscences are simply designed to decay after a particular term. They simply disappear from our brains on the identical time as a positive time period passes during which a person doesn't get proper of access to it. Here, the analogy of a call that is written on sand in the desert works pretty nicely. Just as a call slowly fades away whilst deposits of sand cowl it up, a memory moreover fades away with time. If we preserve cleansing and rewriting the call at the sand, it's going to live intact. Similarly, a memory remains smooth in our thoughts if we hold getting access to it. Otherwise, it clearly decays just like the decision on the sand.

Still, this idea has its vulnerable factors. Some studies advise that the decay concept is a delusion for people due to the fact some reminiscences remain intact in our extended-time period reminiscence for extended durations of time although we don't rehearse them. These memories embody some activities from our childhood that haven't any use for us now and we don't rehearse it, nevertheless we are capable of retrieve it after a passage of 25 years or greater.

Role of Interference

Another precept that subjects lots is the inference concept which suggests that recollections compete and interfere with every different. It takes area whilst memories have similar facts. When interference occurs among reminiscences, they grow to be an awful lot much less available to us. It takes location to college college students on the identical time as they'll be trying to investigate the identical lesson again and again. Let's take a look at out the varieties of interference:

Retroactive interference: It takes area at the same time as new records interferes with our ability to hold the information which we had formerly located out.

Proactive interference: It occurs in our mind at the same time as an antique reminiscence places hurdles for a trendy reminiscence to be stored in our mind. It makes it almost now not possible for a present day memory to find room.

Motivated Forgetfulness

Sometimes, we try to miss our memories deliberately which includes certain traumatic reports and traumatic opinions that we ought to go through. Painful and worrying studies will be predisposed to be pretty frightening and tough for us and moreover push us into deep depression and anxiety. That's why we need to miss the ones studies as speedy as viable.

Chapter 24: Structure and Types of Memory

This financial disaster is going to stroll you via distinctive reminiscence sorts and their function in our mind. Among the ones types are visible, photograph memory, verbal-splendid judgment memory, emotional memory, sensory memory, and spontaneous reminiscence. Unless we don't understand specific reminiscence kinds, we cannot improve them and moreover we can not use them to beautify the storage of records in our brains and additionally we can't be confident in memorizing information.

You may additionally study motor reminiscence which will be very useful in assisting you discover ways to energy a vehicle, a motorbike or a deliver. You can even study distinct subtypes of sensory reminiscence. In addition to losing light on how you could decorate your reminiscence, the bankruptcy will stroll you via the signs of a terrible visual memory.

Visual or Image Memory

Visual reminiscence is defined as a skills that a scholar should need to do properly at any degree in their schooling. It plays a important role in university students' studying. If a pupil has seen reminiscence abilties, he can be terrific at studying new topics and lectures. On the opposite hand, if college college students display off negative visual reminiscence, they'll be possibly to be concerned through perturbed studying in the educational fields. Visual memory is considered as a huge location that is typically known as seen perceptual abilties. It makes a speciality of someone's ability to bear in mind first-rate records as it become visible.

It is a vital detail close to judging our analyzing and writing talents. For instance, whilst a infant gets a preserve of a pocket e-book and a pencil and starts offevolved offevolved writing a word on it, she or he want to keep in mind the formation of diverse components of the letter from their reminiscence. He wants to write the phrase 'snazzy,' he's going to ought to maintain in thoughts wherein formation the 5 letters are in positioned inside the phrase and which letters must be repeated inside the word. Just recall, if he has a inclined visible memory and the images they devise in his thoughts usually generally tend to vanish away short, they'll be extraordinarily annoyed to perform this easy feat of writing.

If a pupil in a category suffers from a vulnerable seen reminiscence, his or her ordinary general overall performance will undergo due to the fact they may be no longer capable of maintain up with the pace of the teacher who's writing at the whiteboard with a marker. The scholar might be inside the center of writing a sentence even as the teacher will erase it to begin a brand new one, definitely because of the fact he's going to war to duplicate the letters from the whiteboard to his notebook. This also results in positive mental issues for the scholar which encompass inferiority complex and strain.

He may also additionally struggle in studying sports activities sports because of comprehension issues. Visual reminiscence has kinds: short-time period seen reminiscence and extended-time period visible reminiscence.

• Short-term visible reminiscence: It is the capability of a scholar to recall tremendous pics in a very brief span of time. For example, a pupil is tested 20 quick photographs and is asked to preserve them in thoughts for a period of 1/2-hour. They are then requested to do not forget them proper now after the half-hour window shuts down. This will show off how robust the scholar's visible memory is. This memory is commonly at paintings at the identical time as a student is copying letters or mathematical equations from the whiteboard to a pocket e book.

• Long-term visible reminiscence: It is the potential of a pupil to bear in mind fine locations or pictures that he or she has taken into consideration in a fantastic term within the past. The time span may be a month or twelve months lengthy. A cook dinner dinner dinner who struggles to guide his or her intern may be because of the truth the put together dinner doesn't have an extraordinary seen memory, therefore they'll be no longer capable of maintain in mind the components of a specific recipe.

Visual memory is regularly not feasible to be detected till a infant reaches faculty wherein his seen memory talents are constantly challenged. Some parents forget about those problems, dubbing them as sluggishness and willful negligence on the part of university students, but that is usually no longer the case. As a determine, you must understand what a infant is meant to do and the manner a infant's reminiscence goes to have an effect on his educational capabilities. Here is a rundown of the obligations which visible reminiscence have an effect on at the same time as a little one is enrolled in college.

• Visual reminiscence affects the reading comprehension of a pupil.

• Visual memory lets in a scholar recollect snap shots of terms she or he sees at the whiteboard.

• Visual memory affects a person's capability to don't forget symbols on a calculator.

• Visual memory permits someone shape a mental image of the alphabet or a entire word. It also lets in them be part of one among a type pictures collectively with an photograph of a horse that can be related to the word 'horse,' so that when the pupil sees the picture of the phrase, the photograph of a horse will run in his mind.

Signs of Poor Visual Memory

A scholar who suffers from terrible visible memory now and again exhibits one or more signs which his dad and mom and instructors must realize. The pupil will exhibit:

• Poor skills in relation to remembering spelling.

• Poor skills at the same time as he has to take a look at and comprehend some factor from a ebook.

• Take longer time in copying some element.

• Trouble in running a calculator.

• Slow handwriting talents.

• Trouble in spotting effective numbers and letters.

Visual memory is considered as just like spatial reminiscence. It lets in us document the quantity of place this is spherical us. Where it differs from spatial reminiscence is the fact that visible memory is at artwork at the same time as we are looking at certain gadgets however now not at a specific area.

Verbal-good judgment Memory

Verbal reminiscence is quite a large concept that refers to memory for presenting records verbally. It is the ability that makes university college students brilliantly inexperienced at university and at particular non-instructional paintings. Verbal reminiscence is our capability to preserve in thoughts what we pay attention or study. Verbal reminiscence is notably crucial as it aids college students in learning efficiently at the university. It includes reading, reading and listening abilities, and furthermore recalling the records whilst it's miles wanted the maximum. Verbal reminiscence and verbal reasoning are interconnected to each specific.

If you want to come upon a pupil who has been laid low with prone verbal memory, search for the symptoms and signs and symptoms and signs and symptoms together with vulnerable abilities to consider reminiscences or each distinct info. So, forgetfulness is a sign of a willing verbal memory. Verbal memory issues look like similar to visual reminiscence or on foot reminiscence issues. That's why you want to the touch the school counselor in case you seem to come upon them for the duration of an goal take a look at or a excellent observation. Also, you can attempt out a verbal memory check that is accomplished with the useful resource of a professional (Verbal Memory: The Key to Learning Efficiency, n.D).

If you want to make verbal reminiscence more efficient, you can adopt plenty of strategies which incorporates dual-coding or repeating in a noisy voice what you've got were given truely look at or discovered through hearing. Repeating it in loud phrases is a useful way to memorize subjects in a concrete way.

Verbal memory takes into consideration recalling of phrases and language-based totally reminiscence. This form of reminiscence is also positioned close to brief-time period memory as it has the functionality to hold statistics in an lively usa for a fast time period. Short-term verbal memory has 3 fundamental additives which embody a capability to keep facts, period of the live of the information inside the reminiscence, and the system of encoding this is critical for converting some detail into lengthy-term reminiscence. It is the method of encoding that allows you to rehearse a bit of data and keep in mind it in some time. (Verbal Memory: The Key to Learning Efficiency, n.D)

Motor Memory

Motor memory is hooked up to motor studying. It revolves across the coordination of our muscular device. There are a couple of examples of motor studying along with using a bicycle, riding a vehicle, gambling violin or gambling tennis. If your son loves video video video games, he's going to by no means forget about a way to carry out a play-station or an Xbox. Our muscle tissue maintain in thoughts this shape of specific coordination.

Motor memory, like any other shape of reminiscence, has prolonged and quick shape components. Short-term motor memory can be very a bargain much like the verbal short-time period reminiscence. Short-term memory shops a piece of facts best for a fast time. If we want to do not forget the machine of doing a project for an prolonged time frame, we will need to replicate the task a couple of times to transport it from quick-time period memory to lengthy-term reminiscence.

Traditional information additionally known as episodic memory starts its journey within the hippocampus location of the mind and concludes the journey inside the cerebral cortex. But, for motor reminiscence, topics are considered one in every of a kind. Its adventure starts from the cerebral cortex. A particular sort of neurons additionally called purkinje neurons are taken into consideration because the supply of the quick-time period reminiscence. Purkinje neurons are answerable for transmission of indicators to the cerebellum, the part of our mind that governs the motion of someone (Brown, 2017).

These unique neurons play an vital function in the conversion of short-term reminiscence into extended-time period memory due to the fact the actions we rehearse in quick-term reminiscence is going to lengthy-time period memory. When it involves motor memory, extended-term reminiscence is tough to pin right down to a unmarried place of the brain. It is difficult to understand and give an explanation for how the indicators are transmitted from the cerebellum region of our mind and impact our coordinated movement. Researchers allude to interneurons that has one precise job it is to transport alerts to distinct neurons inside the mind. Researchers be given as authentic with that interneurons lay out a ground map for movement of incredible elements of our our bodies.